Artful Grieving

of related interest

Seasons of Grief
Creative Interventions to Support Bereaved People
Edited by Claudia Coenen
Foreword by Kenneth J. Doka
ISBN 978 1 83997 486 1
eISBN 978 1 83997 487 8

The Creative Toolkit for Working with Grief and Bereavement
A Practitioner's Guide with Activities and Worksheets
Claudia Coenen
Illustrated by Masha Pimas
ISBN 978 1 78775 146 0
eISBN 978 1 78775 147 7

An Expressive Arts Approach to Healing Loss and Grief
Working Across the Spectrum of Loss with Individuals and Communities
Irene Renzenbrink
Foreword by Stephen K. Levine
ISBN 978 1 78775 278 8
eISBN 978 1 78775 279 5

ARTFUL GRIEVING

50 ART THERAPY DIRECTIVES TO CREATIVELY INSPIRE YOUR PRACTICE WITH GRIEF AND BEREAVEMENT

ALICIA SEYMOUR, MA, ATR-P, NCC

Jessica Kingsley Publishers
London and Philadelphia

First published in Great Britain in 2025 by Jessica Kingsley Publishers
An imprint of John Murray Press

I

Copyright © Alicia Seymour 2025

The right of Alicia Seymour to be identified as the Author of the Work has been
asserted by her in accordance with the Copyright, Designs and Patents Act 1988.

Front cover image source: Alicia Seymour. The cover image is for
illustrative purposes only, and any person featuring is a model.

*Content Warning: This book mentions a variety of circumstances related to
trauma and bereavement, including loss of a loved one, abortion, sexual abuse,
rape, suicide and suicidal ideation, and death from accidents and violence.*

A CIP catalogue record for this title is available from the
British Library and the Library of Congress

ISBN 978 1 80501 369 3
eISBN 978 1 80501 370 9

Printed and bound in the United States by Integrated Books International

Jessica Kingsley Publishers' policy is to use papers that are natural,
renewable and recyclable products and made from wood grown in
sustainable forests. The logging and manufacturing processes are expected
to conform to the environmental regulations of the country of origin.

Jessica Kingsley Publishers
Carmelite House
50 Victoria Embankment
London EC4Y 0DZ

www.jkp.com

John Murray Press
Part of Hodder & Stoughton Limited
An Hachette UK Company

The authorised representative in the EEA is Hachette Ireland,
8 Castlecourt Centre, Dublin 15, D15 XTP3, Ireland (email: info@hbgi.ie)

CONTENTS

ACKNOWLEDGEMENTS

There were many people who influenced and aided this book. First, without Ronnie this book may never have happened. His life impacted mine in ways I'm only now realizing, and his death was the catalyst for my life-changing journey with grief. While our relationship was complicated, loving each other was easy because it was real. I hope he knows how thankful I am for him and that I will always love him.

My friend and colleague Carolyn Brown-Treadon was the first to recognize the value of my work. She supported my first AATA presentation and pushed me forward when I didn't know if I wanted to keep going. I will be forever thankful for her.

I want to thank my friend, colleague, and mentor David Gussak. Not only did Dave see my potential and believe in my work; he generously poured his time and knowledge into helping me clarify my vision and voice. He saw something in me that I didn't always see in myself, and his guidance helped me become a better writer, clinician, and person. Thank you, Dave!

Thank you to all my colleagues and friends for their unwavering support. Their excitement for the book and encouragement meant the world to me. This was not always an easy process, but I was blessed to be surrounded by amazing people.

I want to thank the families who allowed me into their lives during their difficult journey with death. Your honesty, strength, courage, and resilience helped shape this book and my understanding of the complexities of grief. I will be forever grateful to you all.

Finally, I want to thank Chuck and our son, Liam. Only a baby when I went back to graduate school, Liam spent countless hours with me in classes, doing homework, and writing this book. I hope someday he understands the long hours I had to work and how important it was. I am so blessed to be his mom and love him more than I could ever say.

A NOTE BEFORE BEGINNING

Before beginning this exploration of grief, I feel a warning is necessary. The case examples of loss provided may be triggering for some. Those who seek grief counseling are more likely to have experienced elements of trauma related to their loss, which is reflected in the examples. To highlight the complex nature of loss and grief. I felt it necessary to provide honest and oftentimes painful cases. If an example does trigger you, take time to process it. There are many directives in this book that may assist you. Still, if you find yourself overwhelmed by this content, it may be a sign it is time to stop and care for yourself before returning to the material. True and healthy grief work is a combination of work and rest.

PREFACE

In the summer of 2021, as the world entered the newest COVID-19 variant surge, the world was divided into two parts—those that had experienced illness or death of a friend and loved one, and those who had not. I was fortunately part of the latter group. This irrevocably changed on July 18th. As I was scrolling through social media, I saw a post that Ronnie, the man who had been my first love, on-and-off partner, and friend of 23 years, was dead from COVID-19. I had never experienced such loss and remember feeling like I couldn't breathe or stand. While our relationship was far from perfect, I was devastated. I thought about the years of love and pain that I had avoided processing, but any chance of closure and healing seemed to die with him. Possibly the worst part was that I believed I couldn't tell anyone of all that I had gone through and was feeling for fear of judgment and misunderstanding.

At the time, as a graduate student in an art therapy program, I was selecting a site for me to complete my practicum requirements and decided—for ill or for good—the only way to process this and so many other losses was to face death directly. I reached out to a local hospice that was willing to take me on as an intern. With the beginning of the fall semester, I began my work with patients and their families, and I quickly realized that through my own experiences I had much to offer, and my greatest contribution was in grief counseling; this became my primary focus.

During this period, although I have an autoimmune disease, because giving birth to my first child was fairly easy, my then husband and I were attempting to have our second baby. Still, I knew it could be difficult due to my illness, but the doctors thought I had a chance.

After many struggles, it became apparent that not only would a second baby be impossible, but I would also need a total hysterectomy. Within three months my world shattered again.

I was distraught over my lost fertility. My doctor knew I was finishing my graduate studies so she was not surprised when I expressed my desire to have my uterus returned to me so I could make art with her before giving her a proper burial. After the procedure, my uterus was returned, and we made beautiful art together before her funeral. Although this ritual helped, I still felt sad and off in a way I couldn't explain. Then it hit me. I was grieving. Even though I had been diving deeply into the grief literature to inform my professional practices, I had no idea you could grieve a hysterectomy. I erroneously believed that grief was only for a real death, right?

Two weeks after my surgery, I suffered yet another loss. My maternal grandmother had an accident resulting in irreversible damage and was immediately placed in hospice care. Due to my surgery, I was unable to travel to her and could only have one phone call before she died. There was no funeral or memorial as the other family members did not desire such rituals. My last grandparent was just gone.

The surgery, stress of multiple losses, and the demands of graduate school caused a flare of my neuromyelitis optica, the potentially lethal autoimmune disease mentioned above. This particular one causes the immune system to attack the spinal cord. An MRI showed a potentially lethal spinal cord lesion, and I was started on a high dose of chemotherapy and plasmapheresis. On my first day of the treatments, my son contracted COVID-19. I was in denial that I could get it and about how sick I could become; that was until I too got it. As I lay in bed out of my mind with fever and gasping for air, I began to realize I could die this time. I had previous life-threatening moments with my illnesses but had never felt that close to actually dying. As I begged the universe to let me live, I clearly heard someone ask me if I was ready to spend my life walking with death. Although I might have been hallucinating, I answered yes—just in case. Shortly after, my fever broke, and I could breathe again. But I made a promise.

That was the moment when the grief work became a more personal journey of creation and self-discovery. I took what I had learned about grief counseling and compared it to art therapy literature, finding a gap that was discouraging. To address these gaps, I decided to attempt to create new directives based on grief-counseling models. The directives were guided by extensive research in grief, death, spirituality, and trauma, and I began to use them in my work. I quickly saw the positive impact on my clients, both the dying and the bereaved.

With the support of colleagues, I presented the basis for *Artful Grieving* at a national conference (Seymour & Treadon, 2022). The feedback was greater than I had anticipated with attendees expressing a desire for new grief-focused directives that addressed losses of all kinds. My directives appeared to meet their expressed needs, and I was encouraged to turn them into the book you are now reading.

This book became the way I made meaning of so much loss and suffering, both personal and professional. It is my hope that the directives will create new avenues for addressing the potential challenges of grief and for seizing the opportunity for amazing transformation and healing. I hope that my chosen field of art creation, which I love, can be combined with empirically supported grief-counseling models to have the greatest possible impact in our work. Grief is not an enemy to be fought against, but a natural part of life that holds the power to create positive change in a way no other experience can.

CHAPTER 1

GRIEF AND LOSS

Amanda is a 24-year-old woman whose husband died suddenly. She found herself as a young widow and single mother of their two-year-old daughter. Amanda was overwhelmed by the drastic and sudden changes to her life. Her emotions varied from deep sorrow to anger and increasingly long periods of numbness. She became concerned about her ability to adapt to life without her husband.

Andy is a 42-year-old man who was concerned about his increased alcohol consumption. His drinking escalated after his wife suddenly divorced him following 20 years of marriage. Although he acknowledged the relationship had issues, he was shocked when she filed for divorce. His attempts at reconciliation were unsuccessful. He longed for the return of his wife and the life they shared.

Henry, a 50-year-old man, and his wife were involved in a car accident. They were both seriously injured and required hospitalization. Henry recovered, but his wife died after she spent several months in a coma. Henry experienced guilt and shame, not only due to his survival, but also because he felt relief at his wife's passing. He had been warned that if his wife had survived, she would have likely required lifelong care.

Grief is not a clinical diagnosis or anomaly of functioning, but the normal reaction to loss (Worden, 2018). As a universal human response, it occurs across cultures, impacting everyone regardless of race, gender, sexual orientation, or socioeconomic status (Shear, 2012). Loss comes in many forms, including illness, divorce, and death. For most, grief is a normal process that does not require intervention, but for others it can become a chronic condition with far-reaching and potentially lethal consequences (Zisook & Shear, 2009).

"Grief is the anguish experienced after significant loss, usually the death of a beloved person" (American Psychological Association, 2018). This anguish is a combination of emotional and physical reactions to the loss, which may include but are not limited to anger, sadness, blame, guilt, anxiety, loneliness, helplessness, shock, yearning, relief, numbness, desperation, despair, apprehension, apathy, denial, hopelessness, shame, ambivalence, irritability, and depersonalization (Rando, 1984; Worden, 2018). Other reactions may include social withdrawal, difficulty concentrating, sleep disturbances, disordered eating, restlessness, self-punishment, sexual dysfunction (either lack of drive or hypersexuality), and somatic symptoms such as chest pain, fatigue, headaches, and gastrointestinal issues.

Societies and cultures have unspoken but understood guidelines regarding which losses qualify as significant; not all losses or their subsequent grief are considered equal. This leads to inconsistency in recognition and support. The American Psychiatric Association's (2022) diagnostic criteria for Prolonged Grief Disorder is quite limiting; it claims that clinically significant loss only occurs with the death of a "loved one." This discounts the significance of non-death losses or deaths that some may seem as less impactful but in fact can be quite overwhelming, such as the death of a pet; even the death of an abuser can result in extremely complicated and prolonged grief. Such limitations prevent these experiences from being recognized as potentially high risk for clinically significant grief. Without this acknowledgement, appropriate interventions may not be taken, further increasing the likelihood of developing severe complications. Regardless of the limited views by such clinical associations—and, by extension, society—only an individual can determine the significance of their loss (Doka, 2002).

GRIEVING VS. MOURNING

Grieving and *mourning* are terms that are often used interchangeably; however, they have slightly different meanings (Worden, 2018). Grieving typically refers to internal processing, while mourning is the external expression of grief. The literature and popular culture tend to think of mourning in the context of the death loss. Grieving, however, is used to describe the entire reaction and subsequent processing.

To minimize potential disenfranchisement, this book will use *grieving* to describe the full process of grief from all losses. Some may argue that this is not a completely accurate descriptor and that the distinction is necessary; however, this book includes art directives to address not only the internal processing, but also the outward expression of grief with some facilitating both. Using the term *grieving* allows for recognition of both the internal and external aspects of the grief experience while acknowledging the significance of all losses without seeming to place greater importance on a particular type of loss.

ATTACHMENT

The relationship between the bereaved and what or who was lost will often be a predictor of the magnitude of the grief reaction. One lens through which to examine this relationship is through Bowlby's attachment theory (2008). This theory "conceptualizes the tendency in human beings to create strong affectional bonds with others and is a way to understand the strong emotional reaction that occurs when those bonds are threatened or broken" (Worden, 2018, p.15). These attachments start in childhood and are often carried into adulthood, and are distinguished as either secure or insecure, with insecure further categorized as anxious/preoccupied, avoidant/ambivalent, avoidant/dismissive, or avoidant/fearful.

Individuals with secure attachments tend to feel supported and worthy of care (Worden, 2018). When grieving, they are able to process their painful emotions while continuing with their daily activities. They may also create healthy continuing bonds with the deceased and emotional ties after death and feel that those bonds support them in their future.

Insecure attachments, however, are often a result of conflicted or inadequate parental relationships and care. If an anxious/preoccupied attachment is prevalent, the person may feel "uneasy" about the relationship and often show "high levels of distress" when the object of their attachment is lost (Worden, 2018, p.69). They may also experience high levels of helplessness, low self-efficacy, and increased longing for the deceased. In anxious/ambivalent attachments "love and hate coexist on almost equal levels" (p.70). These people may focus on exaggeratedly positive aspects of their relationship to avoid experiencing their heightened anger and anxiety. Without acknowledging both positive and negative, these people may experience increased depression and complicated grief. Those with an avoidant/dismissive attachment often had to rely on themselves, valuing autonomy and self-reliance; thus, their grief reaction may be minimal. The one experiencing an avoidant/fearful attachment may be "very likely the poorest adaptation to the loss" (p.71) due to their fear of broken attachments and losing those they care about. When death severs their relationship, they are more likely to experience higher levels of depression, social withdrawal, and increased difficulty making needed life adjustments. Since attachment is based on a variety of individual personality and relationship factors (Worden, 2018), two people who experienced identical losses would not be expected to experience the same grief reactions. Those with secure attachments would be expected to experience more balanced and healthy grief compared to those with insecure attachments.

The amount a person was loved is not always an indicator of attachment, since even those with insecure attachments may express love for the deceased. For example, if the relationship was conflicted or traumatic, the person may hold on to deep affection and care but will likely experience more intense grief symptoms with greater difficulty processing and making sense of their subsequent loss (Figley, Bride, & Mazza, 1997; Worden, 2018). This may be seen when the deceased was narcissistic or overly dependent, following such a loss, the bereaved may have increased difficulty making needed life adjustments due to previous dependence, low self-esteem, and helplessness.

Kho et al.'s (2015) study on attachment styles and grief responses found that those with anxious attachments showed both greater emotional responses and difficulty accepting the reality of the loss. These findings were reinforced by Russ et al. (2022), who conducted a systematic review of the literature of complicated grief and attachment style. Their review found that individuals with insecure attachments were at greater risk of developing complicated grief, with anxious attachments being consistently at higher risk than those with avoidant attachments.

Understanding the individual's attachment style can give the clinician important insight into their potential grief experience. In cases of insecure attachment, the clinician may be able to address attachment-specific issues early in the therapeutic relationship, such as helping to balance positive and negative emotions or addressing feelings of anger, guilt, and social withdrawal. If the attachment was fearful, steps can be taken to encourage positive social engagement and secure attachment formation in the future. This early intervention may aid effective processing and the prevention of clinically significant grief.

DISENFRANCHISED GRIEF

Tom and Ed had been in a committed relationship for almost 15 years. Without warning, Ed had a heart attack and died. Tom and Ed never married; so, after Ed's passing, his estranged parents—who had never accepted that their son was gay—were called to make the arrangements for his funeral. Tom was told he was not allowed to attend and reported feeling deep hurt and sadness at being excluded from saying goodbye to the man he loved.

Ben is a 27-year-old inmate at a state prison. While he was incarcerated, his girlfriend was murdered by a jealous ex-boyfriend. As she had been his primary support and only visitor, Ben felt that he had lost his hope and ability to cope with the challenges of prison life. Ben experienced intense blame, guilt, anger, and shame that he was unable to protect her due to the consequences of his criminal activities.

> Yuko is a 19-year-old woman who underwent an abortion after a rape. She had always wanted to have children but could not see herself being a mother under these circumstances. She felt intense feelings of guilt and shame for her decision, which was greatly increased when she had to travel to another state to receive the procedure due to restrictive laws in her home state. She experienced self-blame to such an extent that she stopped caring for her basic needs and began to socially isolate from friends and family out of fear that they would learn of her actions and label her a murderer.

The perception of grief and its expected manifestations and outcomes is a product of an individual's culture, social norms, and personal beliefs (Doka, 2002). One function of society is to establish unspoken but understood rules or norms for how individuals are expected to behave in social situations. These norms aid in the functioning of society, but any violation could lead to ostracization. This may be seen when the person experiences a type of loss that is in opposition to the majority, such as in cases of non-death losses. When grief violates social norms, it may be considered disenfranchised or unseen; it becomes a type of "grief that is not openly acknowledged, socially validated, and publicly observed" (Doka, 2002, p.5). Thus, "although the individual grieves, others do not acknowledge that the individual has a *right* to grieve" (p.6, italics added).

Doka (2002) noted several types of grief that were commonly disenfranchised. The first related to unrecognized and "nontraditional relationships—such as extramarital affairs, cohabitation of unmarried people, and homosexual relationships" (pp.10–11). Although unmarried or homosexual relationships have since been more accepted, they may not be considered as valid as the grief of the traditional widow/widower.

Extramarital affairs are almost always seen as unacceptable, with the surviving paramour being a target of anger and blame instead of support and understanding. While their grief may be as intense as the surviving spouse's—especially if the affair had lasted for years—they are often ostracized from grief rituals, forcing them to grieve in isolation. Such affairs, due to their secretive nature, create the potential for insecure attachments (Russell, Baker, & McNulty, 2013), which create even more intense and difficult grief processing. Unfortunately, the literature on the grief experience of the extramarital partner is scant at best, often tending to focus on the grief of the spouse who is aware of the affair. This, in and of itself, is a remnant and reinforcement of the disenfranchisement, creating bias in the researcher.

Another commonly disenfranchised loss is miscarriage (Doka, 2002). The loss of a pregnancy, especially if it is early, is not seen to be as impactful as when someone loses a baby or small child. Miscarriages are often minimized, and a woman's grief is often placated with "Well, you can always try again." This even seems to be endorsed by the medical community, advising women to keep their pregnancies a secret before reaching 12 weeks' gestation (Brier, 1999) as the first 12 weeks are the highest risk for miscarriage. As a result, if they lose the fetus during this period, they are denied the opportunity for social support. A study conducted by Brier (1999) found that women experienced high rates of anger and dissatisfaction with their care after a pregnancy loss, as they felt unsupported and that their doctors did not acknowledge the emotional impact of the loss. If a woman elects to abort her pregnancy, the resultant disenfranchisement may be even more harsh as they are seen as responsible for the loss, regardless of the reason or of the woman's resultant responses (Doka, 2002).

Social death "in which the person is alive but is treated as if dead" is also commonly disenfranchised (Doka, 2002, p.11). An example would be if someone has so radically changed that they are no longer viewed as the same person. This may occur for a variety of reasons, including mental illness, dementia, or substance abuse; the person they knew before is perceived as dead, inducing a radically different kind of grief, one that society often does not acknowledge since the person is still living. This includes those who are incarcerated (Read, 2018), particularly since they are often seen by society as deserving of such loss and punishment. Any grief they or their families experience is considered justified.

The family of the inmate may experience grief due to the loss of their loved one while serving their sentence (Doka, 2002; Read,

2018). The family members mourn not only the person's absence, but any hopes or dreams they had for the incarcerated. They may feel as if society has judged them as responsible for the actions of their loved one, even if they played no part in the criminal activity, creating increased shame and social isolation. Even still, such disenfranchisement does not end after release. The formerly imprisoned are subjected to a lifetime of social death and stigma, creating cycles of ongoing loss and grief.

Disenfranchisement is often applied to individuals who are believed to be "not capable of grief" (Doka, 2002, p.13). This group tends to include children, the elderly, and those with developmental disabilities. In children and the elderly, there may be a belief that they are being protected from the pain of death by being excluded from funerals or memorials, although such exclusion often creates more difficulty. Many in society erroneously believe those with developmental disabilities are unable to understand the grief ritual; yet "people who are developmentally disabled are indeed able to understand the concept of death" and would thus benefit from inclusion in the grieving process (Doka, 2002, p.13).

Often, there are few acceptable methods for the bereaved who are experiencing such disenfranchisement to overcome the unseen nature of their grief, and who are unable to receive the needed support, thus leaving them with no choice but to grieve alone. They often recognize that if they were to express their grief and seek support, they may be blamed, shamed, or invalidated. As a result, they may feel that the potential consequences outweigh the potential benefits, thus choosing to remain silent and consequently exacerbating their normal emotional responses to loss, including guilt, shame, anger, powerlessness, loneliness, and hopelessness.

ANTICIPATORY GRIEF

Mary is a 65-year-old woman who has raised her now 20-year-old grandson since birth. Two years ago, her grandson was involved in a robbery that ended in murder. Although facing life in prison, he was given a bond, released on his recognizance as he cooperated with prosecutors, and in that time started college. Although she had been advised he would still likely face a lengthy prison sentence despite his current actions, life took on the illusion of normalcy and her hope increased. As his sentencing approached, however, Mary experienced anxiety, sleep difficulties, overwhelming sadness, rage, and hopelessness.

Bob's wife Linda received a diagnosis of Lewy body dementia at the age of 62. Bob had noticed Linda becoming increasingly forgetful and angry but blamed himself for her behavior. Linda's declining health and increasing violent outbursts became difficult for him to manage. He refused to send her to a nursing facility because he and Linda had promised to care for each other until the end. Bob experienced deep sadness and fear as he watched the wife he knew and loved die.

Grief does not always begin after a loss has occurred but may start months or years prior. Anticipatory grief is experienced due to an expected loss where a person begins to process emotions in preparation for an impending actual loss. Although seemingly future-focused, such a person may also grieve the past and present as well (Rando, 2000). While occurring in a variety of death and non-death losses, it is most commonly related to a looming death from illness. When someone is diagnosed with a terminal illness, their family may begin to grieve not only the future death of the individual, but also the ongoing losses related to increasing deterioration, which may create social death before their actual demise. These reduced social supports could impact the individual's ability to process their emotions once the death has occurred. Further, since their grief tends to be prolonged, by the time the death occurs, a person may feel that they are burnt out from extended grieving and unable to effectively process the loss.

Anticipatory grief related to dementia has received special attention in the literature (Mittelman, Epstein, & Pierzchala, 2003). Dementia is a general term used to describe illnesses that are marked by decreased memory formation and recall that inhibits functioning. There are a variety of underlying illnesses that may create dementia, such as

Alzheimer's disease. While treatments are available that may slow the underlying condition, most forms are progressive with periods of relative stability followed by sharp declines in memory and physiological functioning. When these declines occur, how severe they may be and how long the stable periods will last cannot be predicted, potentially creating more difficult emotional reactions. The loved one does not know when the next decline will occur, creating even more anxiety and fear. In periods where the patient demonstrates symptom stability, the person may begin to doubt the diagnosis, exacerbating the reactions when the next inevitable decline occurs. Dementia also changes the individual's personality: the once kind and quiet mother now no longer remembers her daughter and reacts with violence and aggression when she sees her. These personality changes may be especially difficult for family and friends; for while their loved one is still technically alive, the person they knew is dead.

This type of grief is not limited to the loved ones of the person who is ill but may also occur for those with a chronic and life-threatening illness themselves (Doka, 2014). These people will grieve the lives they had, their present life that is now focused on declining health and painful treatments, and losing the future life they had hoped for. This pattern of grieving past, present, and future may be a pervasive cycle, heightened during times of disease progression and increased disability.

Anticipatory grief is also seen in the criminal justice system, not only for the accused, but for their families as well, as seen in the example of Mary above (Hunt, 2021; Jones & Beck, 2006). From the time of arrest, the individual and their family may begin to anticipate loss as they await the conclusion of the case and possible sentencing. This wait may drag on for years. For both accused and family, the resultant ambiguity creates a time of living and not living, with decisions based on possible prison sentences instead of personal desires. Whether incarcerated or free on bond, the accused may feel that they are losing their lives as each day passes, unable to move forward until a resolution is reached. Life is overshadowed by the threat of impending loss, creating feelings of guilt, shame, regret, blame, anger, sadness, and hopelessness.

TRAUMATIC GRIEF

Rachel is a 22-year-old woman whose boyfriend was shot and killed during an attempted robbery. Rachel witnessed the event but could do nothing to help her boyfriend except hold him as he died. As time went on, following the traumatic event, she experienced intrusive thoughts, nightmares, and intense fear of public spaces. She was always exhausted due to lack of sleep and began to isolate from family and friends. She refused to move any of her boyfriend's things, explaining that keeping his things made her feel like he would be coming back.

Arjun is a 46-year-old man whose 20-year-old daughter died by suicide. Before her death, she had experienced difficulty adjusting to the demands of college and had chosen to take a semester off to live with her father. Arjun felt his daughter was happy and was shocked to find her deceased after returning home from work. He blamed himself for her death, believing he must have missed the warning signs to get her the help she needed.

Debra is a 35-year-old woman whose grandfather died after a year-long battle with cancer. Debra's grandfather sexually abused her when she was a child. Over time, Debra tried to reconcile the trauma she felt over her grandfather's betrayal while trying to maintain the expected relationship with him as an adult. Debra felt conflicted about the death and her abuse.

While all loss impacts a person's life, not all loss is traumatic (Figley, 2013). Some losses, such as a death that was expected and peaceful or a divorce that was decided upon mutually, are less likely to be considered traumatic. Still, others are more sudden or violent, creating intense emotional responses.

Death from murder is almost always traumatic (Figley, 2013). Murder by its very nature is sudden, violent, violating the norms and laws of society, often leaving a great deal of unfinished business (Worden, 2018). When a young person is killed, it becomes an even greater violation of perceived natural laws, in turn creating more intense spiritual crisis, anger, and guilt. Such a death witnessed by the bereaved often increases the traumatic responses such as flashbacks and intrusive thoughts, compounding the challenges. Any future legal proceedings that often force loved ones to revisit the loss time and time again can often cause new trauma and grief.

Suicide often creates traumatic bereavement (Melhem et al., 2004). Studies reveal increased depression, hopelessness, and difficulty in daily living for those who experienced the loss of a loved one to suicide (Bellini et al., 2018). The surviving family may furthermore experience disenfranchised grief, as ending one's own life is often seen as a violation of social norms and spiritual rules (Doka, 2002). If the deceased and their family were active members of a group that took harsh views against suicide such as a particular church, survivors may feel that they are being judged or blamed for the death. They may experience the withdrawal of previous social support, increased feelings of isolation, stigmatization, guilt, shame, and hopelessness.

Traumatic loss may create more complex and difficult grief (Figley, 2013). Normally occurring fear, guilt, despair, anxiety, sleep disturbances, intrusive thoughts, sadness, and helplessness may become more severe and long-lasting and have greater impact on daily functioning (Worden, 2018). Thus, the traumatized griever may require more specialized and intensive treatment, resulting often in complicated grief.

COMPLICATED GRIEF

Ashley is a 33-year-old woman whose six-month-old baby died from SIDS. In the 11 months since her baby's death, Ashley had become increasingly depressed and hopeless. She refused any affection from her husband and was barely caring for herself, often not eating or bathing for days at a time. She would alternate between extreme insomnia and excessive sleep. She was fired from her job due to poor performance and numerous absences. Ashley isolated herself, refusing to speak with friends or family. As the anniversary of her baby's death approached, her husband became concerned about her apparently declining functioning. When confronted with her husband's concerns, Ashley admitted to considering ways to end her suffering and reunite with her child in the afterlife. Ashley was admitted to an inpatient facility where she was able to focus on her chronic grief and safety concerns.

Complicated grief occurs when grieving has become chronic, creating clinically significant impact on the daily life of the individual (Shear, 2012), when it becomes a serious issue that affects a person mentally, emotional, physically, behaviorally, and spiritually (Mason, Tofthagen, & Buck, 2020). The condition is marked by an increase in intensity of normal grief emotions, such as anxiety, difficulty concentrating, loneliness, longing, desperation, and guilt. It may also impact physical health, with higher reports of sleep disturbances, pain, heart disease, and autoimmune diseases (Zisook & Shear, 2009). A person experiencing such complicated grief may further engage in self-destructive thoughts and behaviors, including substance abuse and, in extreme cases, suicidality.

Complicated grief occurs in approximately 10–15% of those who grieve a death (Mason et al., 2020). While there is no available data on the rate for those who have experienced non-death losses, this does not mean the condition is absent in this group. Such lack of research is possibly the result of a bias that the death loss is more life-altering and significant than the non-death loss. Arguably, by excluding this group, there are potentially large numbers of people who are not receiving early interventions and appropriate treatment.

Considering the impact on daily living and potential lethality of the condition, early identification and intervention are critical. The risk factors for complicated grief are many, and the type of attachment and quality of the relationship the bereaved has with one they have lost may provide an early warning sign (Shear & Shair, 2005; Worden, 2018). For example, if the relationship was with someone who was narcissistic, highly dependent, or ambivalent with increased hostility, the person experiencing the loss may have more difficulty effectively processing their emotions and making needed life adjustments. Other factors that contribute to such complicated processing of the loss include low socioeconomic status, lower educational background, poor health, inadequate coping strategies, lack of social support, previous substance abuse, degree of trauma associated with the loss, and underlying mental health conditions.

Compounding losses—multiple losses over a short period of time—contribute additional risk factors (Worden, 2018). When they happen rapidly, a person is often unable to fully grieve the first loss before experiencing the new loss and grief. The original grief process is interrupted, and current symptoms become exacerbated. This kind of compounding loss was seen on a large scale during the COVID-19 pandemic, where many experienced loss of health, autonomy, employment, relationships and death (Scheinfeld et al., 2021). To compound this even further, healthy grieving was interrupted due to restrictions on public gatherings; people were unable to attend funerals or receive social support.

While complicated grief is not a clinical diagnosis, it is recognized as a detrimental condition. To address chronic and clinically significant grief, Prolonged Grief Disorder (PGD) was added to the DSM-5-TR (American Psychiatric Association, 2022). Similar in manifestation to complicated grief, symptoms of PGD include disbelief of the death, identity disruption, avoidance of reminders of the deceased, emotional numbness, intense loneliness, feeling life has lost meaning, and difficulty with reintegration. For someone to qualify for a diagnosis, they must have experienced the death of a loved one at least 12 months prior. Still, this fails to recognize the intensity and potential complications that may occur from non-death losses or from deaths of people who were not loved ones. While a critical step in acknowledging the potential impact of chronic grief, its limited scope may be potentially disenfranchising.

PRIMARY AND SECONDARY LOSS

Dan is a 22-year-old man who experienced a spinal-cord injury playing college football. He was paralyzed from the waist down and relied on a wheelchair to get around. He experienced anger and hopelessness after his injury but felt he had already grieved his loss and was determined to move on. However, over time Dan started to experience new feelings of loss. His dreams of hiking across Europe, dancing on his wedding day, and playing football with his future children were now unlikely, and he found himself experiencing renewed grief.

Tina is a 36-year-old single mother of three children under the age of ten who was sentenced to five years in prison for a string of thefts. After years of difficulty maintaining employment due to untreated health conditions, Tina turned to theft to provide for her children. She was never violent, always stealing from large stores, and viewed her crimes as a means of survival. In prison, she found herself experiencing deep sorrow, regret, and anger, not only at the loss of her children, but also for the life milestones she would miss.

Loss is not an isolated event, but one that creates a cascading effect where the initial, primary loss triggers a series of secondary losses (van Wielink, Wilhelm, & van Geelen-Merks, 2020). The primary loss is the event that creates the initial grief reaction and is typically concrete and easily identifiable, such as a death or divorce. Secondary losses are a direct result of the primary loss, such as the loss of friend groups after divorce or future plans due to a death. Initially, the scope and impacts of these losses are not always apparent. Usually developing over time, they create ongoing cycles of grief where the individual experiences renewed grief for the original loss and new grief for the recently acknowledged secondary loss.

Dan's initial loss was his spinal-cord injury. He later experienced a series of secondary losses as indicated. In addition to such concrete losses, other, ambiguous ones may arise, including loss of confidence, security, safety, and self-efficacy. Tina not only lost her freedom and her children, but also lost years of school functions, holidays, and actively participating in her children's lives.

Thus, when exploring grief with a client, it is important not only to validate the primary loss, but also to remain vigilant to potentially emerging secondary losses. Since these are not always apparent to the client, they may surprise the person experiencing them as they become increasingly aware of the full scope of their losses. If not addressed, they could create more intense symptoms of grief, becoming a barrier to effective processing (van Wielink et al., 2020).

NON-DEATH LOSS

Aaliyah is a 26-year-old woman who had a hysterectomy after years of endometriosis. Aaliyah had always thought she would have children once she found the right partner, but now she considers these dreams dead. Although she acknowledged that the procedure greatly increased her quality of life, she found herself feeling deep emptiness, sorrow, and anxiety.

Louis is a 42-year-old man whose home was destroyed after a hurricane. Although his home insurance covered all damages, he realized it would not restore the many family heirlooms that were lost, such as several items from his deceased mother that could never be replaced. Louis had been devastated when his mother died several years prior, and he felt losing her cherished possessions was like experiencing her death all over again.

The non-death loss may have some unique challenges when compared to the death loss, often as a result of biases and prejudices (Harris, 2020). How significant a loss is and how it is recognized are products of social norms. Society considers significant losses to be those from a death, but there is clearly a need to "move away from the stereotype of grief as a reaction to death and understand it more fully and holistically as a reaction to any major loss" (Harris, 2020, p.20). When a norm exists that grief is exclusively associated with a death loss, a person who has experienced a non-death loss may not realize they are grieving, even though the impact and subsequent emotional response may be greater than from a death loss. A person may feel confused or conflicted about their emotional reaction, reporting symptoms such as depression or sadness while also doubting and invalidating their own feelings. This could lead to self-disenfranchisement, where a person does not acknowledge their grief, making them less likely to seek appropriate counseling services. Furthermore, if the counselor is not well-trained in grief, they may not see the non-death loss as a potential source of grief and find their treatments to be inadequate and ineffective.

This bias is further seen in grief research and literature as most studies focus on death-related losses. This is beginning to shift, with more recognition being given to the emotional impact of the non-death loss (Harris, 2020); however, outside of grief research itself, studies of life events that could be characterized as non-death loss tend to be inconclusive, generally focusing on specific psychological impacts rather than allowing for the possibility of grief as a causal factor, even when participants say they are grieving.

One example of this bias is seen in studies of the emotional impact of hysterectomy. Such studies often focus on areas of depression, anxiety, and post-traumatic stress disorder with mixed results (e.g., Cooper et al., 2009; Katon et al., 2020; Leppert, Legro, & Kjerulff, 2007; Pinto et al., 2012; Yen et al., 2008), often concluding women are hysterical and are exhibiting exaggerated emotional responses to gain sympathy and attention. Even in studies where participants indicated they were grieving, researchers did not acknowledge their grief as a cause for their exhibiting symptoms. This seemed to result in women who had a hysterectomy being misdiagnosed or ignored completely, potentially placing them at higher risk of complicated grief. While this is only one example of the gap in the literature, it highlights how bias could create such a blind spot.

Illness-related losses may be unacknowledged because the loss often results in greater chance of survival or quality of life (Doka, 2014), such as a mastectomy (Gershfeld-Litvin, 2018). Mastectomies are often conducted to save the life of the woman and can be "corrected" through breast augmentation procedures. While true, it does not negate the loss experienced.

CHOSEN LOSS

Dylan is a 30-year-old man who has struggled with heroin addiction since the sudden death of his mother five years ago. He has based his daily life and social interactions around his drug use.

After a recent arrest, he was ordered to rehab. Even though he knew he needed to abstain from drug use, he also knew he would lose his friends and the comfort of the drug. He reported feeling high levels of anxiety, distress, and sadness.

Suzy is a 48-year-old woman who recently filed for divorce from her abusive husband. After 19 years of marriage and escalating violence, she knew she had to leave him. Even though the divorce was her choice, she reported feeling conflicted emotions of happiness and deep sadness. She experienced intense guilt and longing for the man her husband had been before he became abusive.

Loss is often thought of as an event that is outside of an individual's control, such as a death, medical diagnosis, or natural disaster. When a person has control over their loss, there may be the disenfranchising belief that it will not—or should not—cause grief; however, this is not always accurate. Even though seemingly voluntary, the loss may be the result of feeling as if there were no other choice. Grief may be further disenfranchised if the result of the loss appears to have a positive impact on the individual. While it may be true that the ultimate result is positive, this may not negate the need to grieve. There is a higher risk of disenfranchisement due to social supports applauding the change without acknowledging the loss or its potential grief (Doka, 2002). Suzy's support system may have been so focused on her safety that they did not acknowledge her need to grieve the loss of her husband; especially if the attachment was conflicted and anxious.

Those in addiction recovery may experience multifaceted grief (Bates-Maves, 2020). Since substance abuse is often a result or symptom of complicated grief, it is possible that the addiction began in response to an unprocessed loss. Furthermore, as a person considers a life without their substance, they may experience feelings of anticipatory grief. It is not uncommon for the individual to organize their life around their addiction, often including a support system composed of others who are battling addiction. As recovery begins, the person will likely consider the secondary losses created by their sobriety, including severing relationships with those who continue to use. For some, the secondary losses become a barrier to sobriety as they are unable to cut off unhealthy relationships. A person experiencing such a loss will need to grieve their past, present, and future losses to remain successfully sober.

While grief is a normal, universal reaction to loss it is not a straight line with all people; it is a complex web of interconnecting factors resulting in vastly different emotions and reactions (Worden, 2018). Its exact manifestation for any individual is based on a variety of factors including the type of loss, attachment, and support received. As the included cases show, grief is far more nuanced than what the official American Psychiatric Association's *Diagnostic and Statistical Manual* (2022) would seem to indicate; To underscore the words of Shear, "I have never climbed Mt. Everest, but I sometimes think it would be easier than navigating the pathway through grief" (2012, p.119).

CHAPTER 2

WORDEN'S TASKS OF MOURNING

Grief counseling has been conceptualized in a variety of ways; the most prominent models rely on stages, phases, or tasks (Worden, 2018). All the models that rely on stages vary in the number of them presented, but all include specific emotional responses, such as anger, denial, and acceptance. A potential problem with these types of models is their tendency to be conceived as those grieving progressing along a straight line, with one stage building off another. Although this may not be what the creators of the models intended, they have generally been popularly perceived as such, with the assumption being that everyone progresses through the identified stages in a linear way.

Kübler-Ross (1969) created one of the best-known—and arguably the most popular—model, referred to as the Stages of Grief. If you were to ask a random sample of people what grief processing is, they would likely attempt to describe it in a way that closely resembled this model. Composed of five stages: denial and isolation, anger, bargaining, depression, and acceptance, it attempts to explain the process of grieving from beginning to end. Although the model explains some aspects of grief, it does not describe variations that may occur (Worden, 2018). For many, there is a belief that all people will go through all stages in an orderly fashion, but this is simply untrue and not a requirement of the stages model. Some will not experience certain stages, while others may have experiences beyond the scope of the described stages. There is potential harm if this model is taken too literally. If a person believes this is the 'right' way to grieve and they deviate from this path, they could view their grief as abnormal, creating a situation where the person engages in self-disenfranchisement.

Phase models are similar to those that rely on stages except they may highlight different aspects of the potential grief reaction and are more strictly linear. The phase model *requires* that a person "pass through" one stage before continuing to the next. Stage and phase models are not inclusive of all grief reactions and have the potential to create barriers when a person's grief does not follow the outlined course.

Worden (2018) believed that the stage and phase models of grief were limiting as, again, they tended to focus on a linear progression, often in opposition to true grief processing. Furthermore, he believed the models were too passive in their expectations, namely that a person would progress through a particular phase or stage without specific action. He felt that this could possibly increase feelings of helplessness in the bereaved. He believed that, in comparison, task models empowered the individual to take an active role in their grieving. By emphasizing concrete objectives, this approach is well suited to work with and supplement other goal-oriented counseling models. Worden is not the only clinician to focus on a task model: Doka (2002), Rando (1984), Stroebe and Schut (1999) have endorsed such an approach as well.

My decision to highlight Worden's Tasks of Mourning (2018) arose from my own clinical experience; and the model's four tasks, which I discuss below, were easily adapted to address a wide range of losses, acknowledging the dynamic and diverse nature of grief. Although Worden, like other grief theorists, was concerned with the death loss, the tasks were still relevant and easily adapted to the non-death experiences. They were practical and useful in a variety of clinical scenarios while minimizing risk of disenfranchisement. It was for these reasons the art directives in this book were based on Worden's model.

TASK I: TO ACCEPT THE REALITY OF THE DEATH

Worden's first task is to accept the reality of the loss by accepting that what has been lost is forever gone. If a person experiences denial and refuses to accept that their loss is permanent, the necessary grieving process may be hindered. Such denial may range from "slight distortion to full-blown delusion" (Worden, 2018, p.42), and could potentially manifest as "mummification"; where the bereaved keeps the deceased's possessions in the state they were in at the time of death. For example, the deceased's bedroom may remain exactly as it was when they died. In extreme cases, this could even include allowing garbage to rot in place. This may frequently be seen in parents who suddenly lose their child.

At the opposite end of this continuum, the person grieving may remove all belongings of the deceased in an attempt to avoid any reminder of their loss. This may also occur in non-death experiences. For example, a person diagnosed with a disabling illness may immediately discard all their sports equipment to avoid reminders of their former life.

Successfully grieving such loss relies on both an intellectual and emotional acceptance (Worden, 2018). The individual must not only rationally accept that the loss has occurred, but they must also feel its emotional impact. Rituals such as traditional funerals or spiritual processes may facilitate this acceptance.

TASK II: TO PROCESS THE PAIN OF GRIEF

Worden's second task requires the person to process the "pain of grief." The word pain is used to describe the entire range of emotional reactions to the loss, recognizing the specificity of its manifestation, intensity, and duration to the individual, often based on the person's attachment to what was lost. A potential barrier to this task occurs when someone is unprepared for the intensity of their emotional reaction. Those with poor emotion regulation or ineffective coping mechanisms may find themselves so overwhelmed that they attempt to avoid and suppress their feelings to maintain functioning. Some avoidance and numbing strategies include abusing substances or working to excess. Although temporarily effective, such strategies could create greater emotional responses when the person is without such crutches.

The well-intentioned but invalidating comments from social

supports may also create emotional blocks (Worden, 2018). When someone experiences a loss, those around them may not know how to react or interact with the grieving person. In an attempt to be comforting they may unwittingly say things that minimize the griever's response. For example, people may make comments about God having a reason for this loss. This may make the person feel that their emotions are contrary to God's intent, potentially, resulting in a heightened spiritual crisis. Others may be chastised for their reactions and encouraged to "cheer up," especially if the loss occurred in the distant past. Such misguided comments often encourage avoidance rather than acceptance of their necessary grief processes. When a person does not feel the pain of their loss, they may enter a state of "not feeling"; this is when they become emotionally numb not only to the loss, but eventually to the world around them (Worden, 2018, p.45). They may engage in "thought-stopping procedures" where they refuse to consider any negative feelings, only wanting and striving to engage in pleasurable thoughts and memories (p.46).

Without processing their powerful emotional responses, a person is at risk of carrying the pain of the loss indefinitely. This pain could become more intense with time, creating an ever-increasing cycle, alternating between feeling pain and wanting to numb it, only to experience it more intensely the next time. To maintain their baseline of numbness often requires an increase in maladaptive behaviors. Experiencing the emotional responses to grief is a critical step in effective processing and minimization of potential harm.

TASK III: TO ADJUST TO A WORLD WITHOUT THE DECEASED

Task III requires an individual to make needed life adjustments after their loss. Worden proposes three such areas: the first, external adjustments, relates to the practical aspects of daily functioning. What or who was lost played a specific role in the life of the bereaved. Those empty roles must now be filled by either the individual themselves or someone else. The second area refers to the internal adjustments related to sense of self, including self-esteem, self-concept, and self-efficacy, all critical for effective grieving. The third adjustment relates to spirituality and worldview. Loss "can challenge one's fundamental life values and philosophical beliefs," which may create a spiritual crisis (Worden, 2018, p.49). The world before loss may have felt predictable, safe, and benevolent; loss, especially if sudden or traumatic, may leave a person questioning their previously held beliefs, which in turn may lead to insecurities, social withdrawal, or hopelessness.

If this task is interrupted, a person may have difficulty progressing through life, often endorsing increased feelings of helplessness (Worden, 2018). While most people adapt to life after loss, the quality and extent of these adjustments will vary, with some people addressing all aspects, while others may only make minimal adjustments as needed. A person's ability to make positive adjustments is critical for future functioning and quality of life.

TASK IV: TO FIND A WAY TO REMEMBER THE DECEASED WHILE EMBARKING ON THE REST OF ONE'S JOURNEY THROUGH LIFE

The final task challenges the individual to find a way to remember what was lost while still moving forward with their own lives. The person or thing that was lost had an impact on the individual, for better or worse. By assessing what this impact was, a person can appropriately place the loss within the greater context of their lives.

In the early years of grief counseling, it was believed that effective grieving could only occur when the bereaved engaged in complete emotional withdrawal from the deceased (Freud, 2005; Worden, 2018). It was soon understood that not only was this task impossible, but it could also be potentially harmful. Currently the value of feeling a continued connection with who or what was lost is viewed as beneficial to a person's ability not only to grieve, but also to move forward successfully. Staying connected with the deceased could take several forms, including talking to the dead, dreaming of them, or honoring them during holidays and transitional ceremonies such as weddings, graduations, or confirmations. This connection may reduce the overwhelming feelings of the permanence of such loss.

When a person struggles with this task, they enter a state of "not living" (Worden, 2018, p. 52). In these cases, the individual is stuck in their overwhelming grief and cannot continue moving forward with their lives. They may experience levels of hopelessness that make them feel any action they take is meaningless, so they choose to take no action. As Worden stressed, "task IV is the most difficult one to accomplish" (p.53).

TASK ORDER AND USE

A common misconception about the Tasks of Mourning is the order in which they are meant to be addressed (Worden, 2018). Due to the numbering of the tasks, people accept this to mean that they must be taken on in a sequential manner. This is incorrect. The tasks are meant to be addressed in the order of client need. Not every person will struggle with the same tasks, and many will address multiple tasks simultaneously. If the impact of the loss had severe consequences on the functioning of an individual's life, they may need to address urgent life adjustments before being able to process the emotional pain of the loss. Others may be able to easily make the needed life adjustments and accept the loss without allowing themselves to process their emotional pain.

For example, consider the person in a car accident that resulted in paralysis. Before attempting to emotionally process their loss they would most likely need to adjust to their new limitations. The adjustments would be paramount to their survival and thus more critical than emotional processing. How would they care for themselves? Would they need to move to a new home that is accessible? Would they need to hire nurses? Once their survival needs are addressed, they would be more likely be able to engage in the emotional processing and acceptance of their loss.

When a person will address a particular task and how much assistance they will need is based solely on the individual (Worden, 2018). Again, grief is not a straight line, and the tasks are meant to be fluid and adaptable to address where the individual is in their grieving process. Further, the tasks were not intended to be addressed only once and then forgotten. Since each task contains many possible elements, a person may need to return to a previously addressed task multiple times to accomplish their specific goals.

While there are a variety of models that attempt to explain grief and its processing, Worden's Tasks of Mourning (2018) stands apart. Its acknowledgment of the diverse and unique nature of grief and ability to adapt to individual needs makes it ideal when working with diverse populations. By requiring the active participation of the client, it works well with other goal-oriented counseling models, striving to increase feelings of power and control to those who may feel helpless in the face of devastating loss.

CHAPTER 3

ART THERAPY AND GRIEF

Before developing the written word, artistic creation was used to communicate ideas, stories, and critical information for survival (Morriss-Kay, 2010). The ability to use symbolic expression is considered by many to be the mark of humanity and consciousness. Art told stories of life and death by representing spiritual beliefs and the journey of the soul. Early people honored their dead through burials that often included art to accompany them into the afterlife. There seems to have been a natural pull toward artistic expression in relation to death and loss, one that has continued through the ages ranging from simplistic to elaborate.

It could be argued that art therapy has tapped into this innate human need for artistic expression to aid healing. By working as a trained guide, the art therapist helps unlock what an individual already understands on a deeper level: that there are times when only art creation can express the depth of their emotions. Continuing a tradition that stretches back to the dawn of humanity, art therapy seems to be a natural choice for helping the bereaved express and process the depth of their grief.

ART THERAPY AS GRIEF RITUAL

In grief counseling, it is often noted that rituals are a needed element of effective grieving (Doka, 2002; Rando, 1984; Worden, 2018), as they are the "highly symbolic acts that confer transcendental significance and meaning on certain life events or experiences" (Doka, 2002, p.135). Such rituals are often used to acknowledge transitions where a person moves from one identity into another.

Death and grief rituals are typically thought of as funerals, celebrations of life, or memorial services (Doka, 2002). These rituals help the bereaved accept the reality of the loss, express emotional pain, and receive social support and connection (Worden, 2018). Unfortunately, needed rituals are not available to all bereaved individuals or considered acceptable for all losses (Doka, 2002). In cases of disenfranchised grief, the bereaved may be excluded. In the non-death loss, there may not be the cultural recognition to mark the transition. In these cases, an alternative ritual may be needed.

When creating alternative rituals, there must be an understanding of what an effective one is. While many have discussed ritual in grief work, Rando (1984) emphasized that ritual properties should meet the therapeutic needs of the grieving individual. Rando's guidance can become a framework with which new activities could be created to meet the needs of the bereaved when more traditional rituals are unavailable.

Rando (1984) noted three therapeutic properties needed for an effective grief ritual. The first was that a ritual must allow the person to experience the "power of acting-out" (p.105). This is a physical action that helps the griever regain a sense of control after their loss. It works by circumventing any intellectual resistance towards experiencing the pain of grief. She further noted, "the physical reality of the ritual behavior touches upon the griever's unconscious feelings *far more effectively than any words can*" (p.105, italics added). The effective grief ritual enables physical expression and action to help empower the client and reduce feelings of helplessness.

The second property is that the ritual must allow for "legitimization of emotional and physical ventilation" (Rando, 1984, p.105). This element is met by giving the griever "permission to outwardly express" their emotions. To meet this need, the ritual must provide "acceptable outlets and *symbols* to focus on" (p.105, italics added). An alternative ritual must provide a space that facilitates the outward emotional expression of grief and channels those feelings into productive endeavors. While verbal processing is an important aspect of grief work, there are populations who may be unable to express themselves verbally. Through using symbolic creation, a person can communicate feelings without the need for words; this may be necessary when a person is nonverbal due to trauma or physiological complications, such as in cases of autism or aphasia. In certain settings, such as prisons, where verbal expression may be limited for safety concerns (Gussak, 2019), symbolism allows grief to be outwardly expressed through coded images that are not easily understood by an outsider, thus providing an element of privacy and protection.

The experience of grief may at times feel overwhelming and all-consuming; the third therapeutic property is that the ritual should allow for the "delimitation of grief" (Rando, 1984, p.105). "Ritual can channel feelings of grief into a circumscribed activity having a distinct beginning and ending with a clear purpose" (p.105), thus allowing the emotions of grief to be more manageable. The efficacious grief ritual provides a container in which the griever has a set time in which they will address a specific area of their grief.

When all three therapeutic properties are considered together, it becomes clear that art therapy is well suited to help facilitate an alternative grief ritual. Occurring in the confines of the therapy session, art therapy is a physical act of creation that uses symbolism to communicate emotions in a productive way. It easily meets all the requirements described by Rando in a way that traditional grief counseling may not, thus arguably making it a needed addition to traditional models.

CURRENT USE OF ART THERAPY IN GRIEF WORK

Art therapists attempt to meet the challenging needs of grief with knowledge gained from grief-focused art therapy literature. Yet the literature offered may be somewhat limited and even formulaic at times. Suggested directives often focus on three main areas of grief: meaning making, memorialization, and continuing the bonds with the deceased (Weiskittle & Gramling, 2018). While such directives are important, particularly as a scaffolding on which to build, they seem to rely on an incomplete view of this dynamic experience. Furthermore, these directives are often offered as standalone exercises with minimal regard to the ongoing complexity and need for layered interventions. With seemingly inconclusive justification for the specific intervention offered, there is little or no explanation for how and why it may be effective in mitigating complex grief. For example, it is often suggested that those who are grieving complete a memory box (Bolton, 2008; Larson, 2017; Potash & Handel, 2012; Rogers & Feldman, 2007; Thompson & Neimeyer, 2014; Young & Garrard, 2015). It has even been featured on *Sesame Street* as an effective, efficient and "widely used" way of addressing memorialization, meaning making, and continuing bonds (Potash & Handel, 2012, p.246).

While indeed popular, and seemingly effective in the short term, the memory box has limitations. First, it is "less appropriate when the bereaved are preoccupied with the post-traumatic symptoms or profound guilt following a violent or problematic loss" (Potash & Handel, 2012, p.243). This limits its effectiveness to only those grieving individuals that had more secure attachments and non-traumatic losses. Often, directives encourage the bereaved to decorate the box with inspirational messages or pictures of the deceased. They are then asked to place mementos into the box to allow for future reminiscing. This may be unintentionally disenfranchising to those experiencing difficult or complicated grieving without high levels of guilt or post-traumatic symptoms (Doka, 2002; Figley, 2013; Rando, 1984; Worden, 2018). Thus, while the memory box may indeed be beneficial for certain types of grief, it could potentially exacerbate negative responses and emotional reactions for those with more complex or even adversarial relationships with the deceased. Other art interventions that focus on memorialization may have the same concerns and limitations as the memory box.

For many, meaning making after loss is a critical aspect of their overall processing (Neimeyer, 2001; Worden, 2018). Loss has the potential to radically change a person's beliefs about the world and their place in it. By finding meaning in the loss, a person may be able to more easily restructure their worldview in a positive and supportive way. Art therapy directives that focus solely on meaning making, while limited, could be beneficial in helping the client begin to assign meaning and restructure worldview.

Art therapy directives that focus on meaning making may be limited when the full process of grieving is taken into consideration. One potential issue is when meaning making is combined with memorialization or continuing bonds. As noted by Weiskittle and Gramling (2018) in a systematic review of 27 studies concerned with grief and art therapy, 11 focused on meaning making of which seven of those also focused on continuing bonds. The review did not note the element of memorialization. In situations where meaning making is combined with continuing bonds or memorialization, the client may feel that their meaning after loss is based on the deceased, implying their locus of control is external. Helplessness and powerlessness are potential barriers to effective grieving; by engaging in artistic creation that emphasizes bonding and memorialization as part of assigning meaning for the self, there is the potential to increase negative self-beliefs. There are certainly art therapy directives that are focused on the internal for meaning making (e.g., Van Lith, 2014); but for others it appears that meaning making has become synonymous with memorialization (Beaumont, 2013). I would further argue that the concept of an art therapy directive being specifically focused on meaning making is based on the fallacy that meaning making is a singular event. Meaning making occurs naturally from consideration of not only the loss, but also its impact on the entire life of the bereaved. This kind of meaning can only occur as grief is processed, becoming a product of the entire act of grieving and not a singular event.

Even those art therapy processes that are designed for non-death-related losses are limited in scope (MacWilliam, 2017). For example, Caruso-Teresi (2017) explored the grief of those who have had a hysterectomy. By developing a curriculum of three art therapy directives, the impact that such a loss may have particularly on the associated changes in the female identity after surgery were elevated. The three directives were informed through a Jungian lens, in particular his archetypes, and included: create a mandala, an archetypal box, similar to the memory box described above, and a clay vessel or pot. Again, while effective for some, requesting the one experiencing such a loss to simply create a clay pot—implying but not necessarily explaining that in doing so they are in effect creating a symbol, a stand-in, for the lost uterus—could be problematic. Such a directive does not take into account those whose grief is so complex that they may react to this creation as reinforcing a counter-intuitive and unhealthy notion that they are not complete without their uterus, and thus have to create an external vessel to replace it and "become whole again." While potentially effective, it is just as likely that this technique could further complicate grieving by increasing feelings of guilt, blame, shame, longing, and sadness, in turn decreasing self-esteem and self-efficacy (Doka, 2014).

Grief-focused art therapy directives, and art therapy directives in general, are potentially further limited by their detailed material lists. One of the hallmarks of being an art therapist is the specialized training and clinical knowledge to use materials in ways that are appropriate and beneficial to the client. The Expressive Therapies Continuum (Hinz, 2020; Kagin & Lusebrink, 1979; Lusebrink, 1987) is one framework used to invoke or inhibit the needed emotional response created by particular art materials. As noted by Gussak (2015), "Art therapists can control the direction of a session by assigning a directive *and the materials to be used*" (p.28, italics added); furthermore, if inappropriate materials are selected, potential harm could be caused by creating unintended "emotional and affective responses [because]certain pathologies do not mix well with certain materials" (p.28). Directives may limit the art therapist's clinical knowledge by offering restrictive and detailed lists of materials to be used often without support for their selections. As noted by Garti and Bat Or (2019), the art medium was "a space in which grief work occurs" (p.196). By restricting material usage in a specific directive, the client's grief work and the specialized training of the art therapist is constricted. Some could argue, wrongly but not without merit, that such directives make the art therapist unnecessary. By providing detailed material lists and specific step-by-step creation instruction, the clinical skill and art of the art therapist is reduced in such a way that gives the impression, without recognizing the potential harm, that anyone could conduct art therapy sessions. This harm may become an even greater concern in cases where there is a heightened risk of complicated grief.

Art therapy allows for symbolic expression and processing of emotion without requiring verbal communication. As noted above, this form of communication may be necessary in situations where verbalization is limited due to medical conditions or safety concerns. When possible, grief work benefits from the combination of verbal and nonverbal expression and processing. Garti and Bat Or (2019) found that art therapists specializing in grief expressed the need for both verbal processing and art creation with some sessions focusing only on verbal elements with no art creation. Current grief art therapy directives often focus on the art creation while providing limited or no processing prompts. Some directives provide minute-by-minute session schedules reducing verbal processing to "ten minutes of art process" without justifying such time limitations (Caruso-Teresi, 2017, p.303). By discussing the image created, the client and clinician gain new insight into the individual's grief and functioning that may facilitate treatment planning.

CHAPTER 4

ABOUT THE DIRECTIVES

This book aims to give the clinician directives/processes that meet the potential needs of the adult grieving client. These directives were not created with the grieving child in mind, and their effectiveness or appropriateness with this group is unknown. I strongly encourage clinicians to review all the directives before using them to allow for suitable selection and, if needed, adjustments in planned session focus. To underscore, this is not meant to provide manualized therapy, as the intuition, judgment, and experience of the clinician could not possibly be reduced to a step-by-step guidebook. The directives are a tool to assist, but not replace, the knowledge of the therapist; it is simply not a recipe book.

The following directives strive to address the limitations present in current grief-focused art therapy practices. To address and change these limitations, it was necessary to alter some common practices in the presentation of directives. Unlike other directives or curriculums, there is no order to the provided interventions. There is no list of suggested weekly assignments for each type of loss. Grief is too individualized. The order in which directives are used will be completely dependent on your client's grief and your clinical intuition. In a general sense, the directives are organized with those addressing emotional reactions or beliefs listed first, followed by relationship and spiritual concerns, and finally those that focus on increasing self-efficacy and future life planning. If there is a struggle on where to begin, I would suggest the processes entitled *Grief Belief* and *My Grief* may be a good way to start the exploration. As any individual client will seldom need all the directives, decisions on which directives to implement should be based on the client and their specific concerns and needs.

While many current art therapy directives list specific materials, most directives included in this book provide a list of general art supplies. The generality allows for the intuition of the art therapist to guide what materials would be most appropriate. There are some directives that need more specific materials, but the art therapist is free to adjust this list without concern for impacting overall effectiveness. This further makes the directives only as expensive as one's budget, allowing selection to be based on need and availability of materials.

Instruction on art completion is purposefully vague and may at times appear redundant. The repetition of instruction is necessary as each directive can both stand alone and work with all other directives. It cannot be assumed that all processes have been considered before selection, so repeating directions ensures consistency. Leaving art creation instruction focused on the topic at hand, instead of on how the client creates the art, encourages unrestricted individual freedom of expression. Overly detailed directions could unintentionally bias the client and possibly create disenfranchisement. For example, if the client were asked to create a collage about a happy memory with the deceased, they may feel that the negative memories they need to express are invalid. The goal is to allow the client's needs to come through their creations without being influenced by the directive or the clinician. If the client is struggling with where to begin, asking them to engage in a visualization exercise may be beneficial.

In contrast with some art therapy directives, there are no time limits in the session descriptions as I find this to be restrictive to creativity and not always in alignment with the needs of the client. Additionally, for newer art therapists there may be a belief that the time limits must be followed exactly. This could distract from the client's needs as the therapist attempts to do the directive the 'right way'. My goal is to allow the clinician to focus on the client and not the clock.

Each directive contains processing prompts to help the client move from discussing the art created to reflection of the topic's greater impact on their lives and how they can continue to move forward into their future. This verbal processing is a critical element of the full directive. It allows for the blending of art therapy and grief counseling techniques to facilitate efficient processing and reintegration. Furthermore, the verbal processing prompts encourage the client to dialogue with their art, possibly allowing them to gain deeper insight into their needs and aid in problem-solving. The provided prompts are merely suggestions to begin the conversation and are not meant to be used as a checklist of questions. In situations where clients do not feel comfortable or are unable to verbally process the work, questions are easily adapted to journal prompts which may be completed as homework and discussed during a following session.

The processes provided are based primarily on Worden's Tasks of Mourning (2018), but also include elements of Stroebe and Schut's Dual-Process Model (1999), cognitive behavioral therapy (Beck & Beck, 2011), dialectical behavioral therapy (Linehan, 2017), solution-focused therapy (Macdonald, 2011), humanism (Schneider et al., 2015), existentialism (Yalom, 1980), ecotherapy (Buzzell & Chalquist, 2009), thanatology (Servaty-Seib & Chapple, 2021), and various forms of spirituality. By drawing from a range of models, directives attempt to address the many possible elements that could arise when working with grief and the methodologies frequently used in clinical practice. Each directive states what task(s) it is addressing and what the goal of the intervention is. This was done to not only provide justification for the directive, but also to allow for easier clinical note taking.

Directives are not limited to individual counseling and may be beneficial to grief-focused groups as well. For groups that are concerned with similar losses, such as death (child, parent, suicide, overdose, murder), health diagnoses, or life transitions, a selection of processes could be compiled to address specific group needs. The interventions to be used and the order with which they are presented would be decided by the clinician based on the group's makeup and needs.

The interventions in this book are intended for both the death and non-death loss. Some directives are worded towards the death loss, but this wording can be easily changed to meet the needs of the non-death ones as well. It was my goal to minimize bias in wording and instruction, allowing for the greatest use and potential impact. Directives are intended to assist the client who is experiencing either normal grieving or is at risk of developing complicated grief. It is not intended for use in the treatment of those who have been diagnosed with complicated grief, which requires a more intensive therapeutic approach that addresses its potentially life-threatening consequences (Worden, 2018). That is not to say that a trained clinician couldn't adapt or add these directives to their practice, but this would only be appropriate for those specifically trained in the condition. If a client is suspected as experiencing complicated grief, the clinician should consider further assessment and referral to more intensive treatment.

ABOUT THE ARTWORK

I created all the included response artwork primarily focusing on my grief from the death of Ronnie, my NMO flare, and hysterectomy, as discussed in the Preface. The art is a raw, emotional, and honest window into my processing. While I never imagined that I would be sharing such deeply personal creations in a book, I included them to provide an example of a real response to the process. Art examples included in other clinical articles and books are typically accompanied by an explanation of the piece. I have not provided such an explanation because I didn't want the story of the work to distract from the directive; however, I think a discussion of the materials I used and some of my processes will be beneficial.

Material selection was based on my clinical knowledge and personal needs. For example, I found that collage materials provided structure for overwhelming emotions while fluid paints allowed greater feeling when emotions were blocked. There were times I used nontraditional materials, such as my own uterus and leftover blood from medical procedures. While some may find this grotesque at first, this was not my intention. I needed to reclaim my power by turning a dark, ugly experience into something beautiful. I wanted the pieces to include me, and I might have taken that desire more literally than others.

My material choices should not give the impression that there are 'correct materials' to use. The materials I selected for the examples may not be appropriate for your clients. As with the directives themselves, clinical intuition and client needs should always guide material usage.

THE DIRECTIVES

GRIEF BELIEF

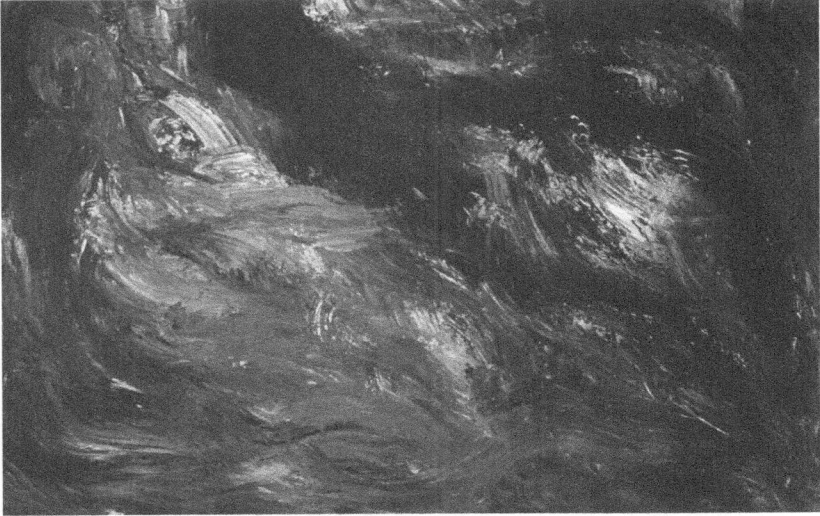

Figure 1: Grief Belief

PURPOSE

Everyone's grief is unique. A person conceptualizes and processes it based on their culture, family, life experiences, and beliefs (Worden, 2018). Feelings about what grief *should* look like are often examined through a cultural lens, creating cognitive distortions (Linehan, 2017) and unconscious bias (Nordell, 2021), which may potentially impede a healthy grieving process. To effectively grieve, it is necessary to explore these biases and their effects with the client.

To walk the path alongside a grieving client, it is critical to first understand their beliefs so that we are speaking the same language. A person may hold beliefs that cause them to unintentionally disenfranchise their own grief, potentially placing them at risk of complicated grief (Doka, 2002). This may include believing that their grieving should be limited in its emotional responses, follow a specific course, or last for only so long. Others may believe grief is only associated with death, unaware or unwilling to acknowledge that they may also grieve another type of loss.

This process focuses on the client developing a macro view of grief. It is possible for their views about the grief of others to be different than their views of their own grief (Doka, 2002). It can be helpful to explore both sides of grief with a client by using both this directive and the following directive, *My Grief*.

Exploring and conceptualizing thought distortions and/or biases through our creation allows them to be challenged (Rosal, 2018), potentially providing new—and possibly more accurate—views of grief. These new perspectives may allow the client to grieve in a more productive way.

GOAL

This process addresses the 1st Task of Mourning. Its goal is to help the client examine their beliefs about the grieving process and any thought distortions and/or biases they may have. Exploring their beliefs can challenge these distorted thoughts, conceptualize specific needs, and allow for goal formation.

MATERIALS

Paper or canvas	Crayons
Paint	Magazine/book clippings
Markers/pens	Scissors
Color pencils	Glue
Pastels	Clay/Model Magic

INSTRUCTION

Ask the client to take a few moments to think about grief. What is grief? How do they feel about grief? Why do they believe people grieve? What does grief look like? What are the "rules" of grief? Ask them to consider how these beliefs are guiding them on their current grief journey. When they are ready, ask them to create a piece that expresses their beliefs about grief and the grieving process.

POSSIBLE PROCESSING QUESTIONS AND PROMPTS

After your client completes their piece, ask them to carefully observe their work and the beliefs that shaped its creation. The following questions may be used to further explore the process.

1. Can you tell me about your work and how it expresses your views on grief?

2. If I asked you, "What is grief?" what would you say?

3. What are your beliefs about the "rules" of grief? Do you think people should behave a certain way when they are grieving? Do you think grief has a time limit?

4. How do you see these beliefs in your own grieving?

5. If you had to sum up your feelings about grief in one word, what would that word be? Why?

6. Are there any thoughts you feel are accurate? Inaccurate? Which ones and why?

7. Are there any beliefs you have that you find helpful? Harmful? Why?

8. Are there any thoughts you would like to change? Which ones? Why?

9. How do you think changing your thoughts about grief would change your grieving process?

MY GRIEF

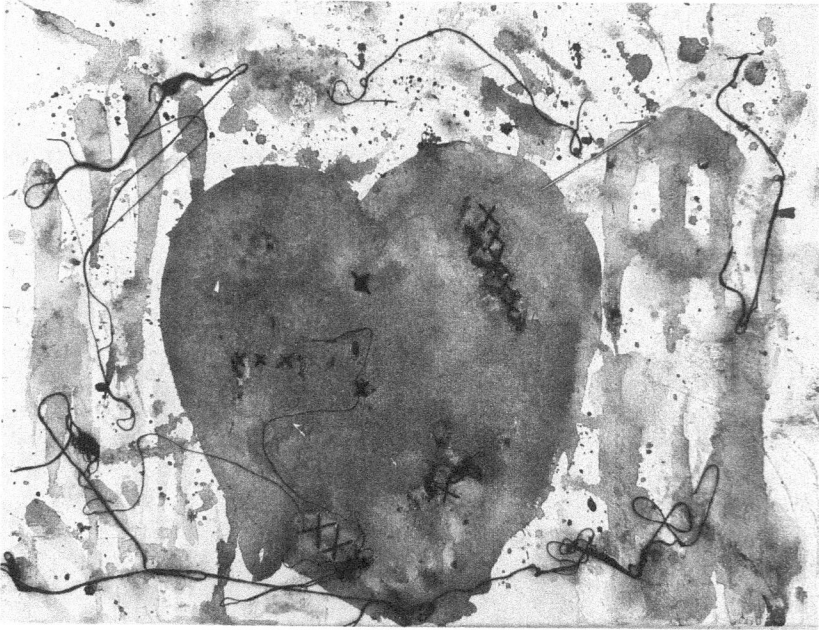

Figure 2: My Grief

PURPOSE

Oftentimes, someone may take a more compassionate and understanding view of grief in others than they do in themselves (Doka, 2002), unaware that they have set higher expectations for themselves. These higher personal standards may create a situation where they unknowingly disenfranchise their own grief. They may begin to see their grief as invalid and unworthy, feeling that their own emotional reactions are inappropriate or abnormal.

Such self-disenfranchisement may create barriers to effective grieving (Doka, 2002). The individual may have a more difficult time processing their emotions and choose to engage in avoidant behaviors, such as closing off their feelings, substance use/

abuse, or overwork (Worden, 2018). While these strategies may feel better in the short term, they can create an increased risk of complicated grief.

A person may not be aware that such behaviors are impeding their own grief (Worden, 2018). By making these known to their clients and providing opportunities for reflection, clinicians are providing them with a critical step in understanding what they need to effectively process their grief, thus allowing for goal formation and future session planning.

GOAL

This process addresses the 1st and 2nd Task of Mourning. Its goal is to help the client analyze how they perceive and explore the idea of grief as something separate with a voice of its own. Such conceptualization can assist them with better understanding their specific needs and the impact of their grief, and with forming goals and action plans to address their needs.

MATERIALS

Paper or canvas	Crayons
Paint	Magazine/book clippings
Markers/pens	Scissors
Color pencils	Glue
Pastels	Clay/Model Magic

INSTRUCTION

Ask the client to take a few moments to think about their grief. What does their grief look like? Feel like? Ask that they imagine their grief as a unique entity with needs and a voice of its own. What is it trying to say? How is it impacting them? How are they interacting with their grief? When they are ready, ask the client to create an image of their grief, how it feels, and what it is trying to say to them.

POSSIBLE PROCESSING QUESTIONS AND PROMPTS

After your client completes their piece, ask them to take time to observe and reflect on their creation. The following questions may be used to further explore the process.

1. Can you tell me about your art and how it reflects your experience?

2. Are there any parts of your creation that stand out to you? Why?

3. How do you view your relationship with grief?

4. If your grief could talk, what would it say? What would you say to it?

5. Was there anything your discovered by creating this piece? If so, what did you discover?

6. How does seeing this work make you feel about your experience? Have your feelings changed?

7. If your feelings have changed, how do you think this discovery will change how you relate to or view your grief?

8. What does your grief need? Want?

9. What actions do you currently take to meet these needs?

10. What actions could you take to meet your needs in the future?

PREVIOUS COPING

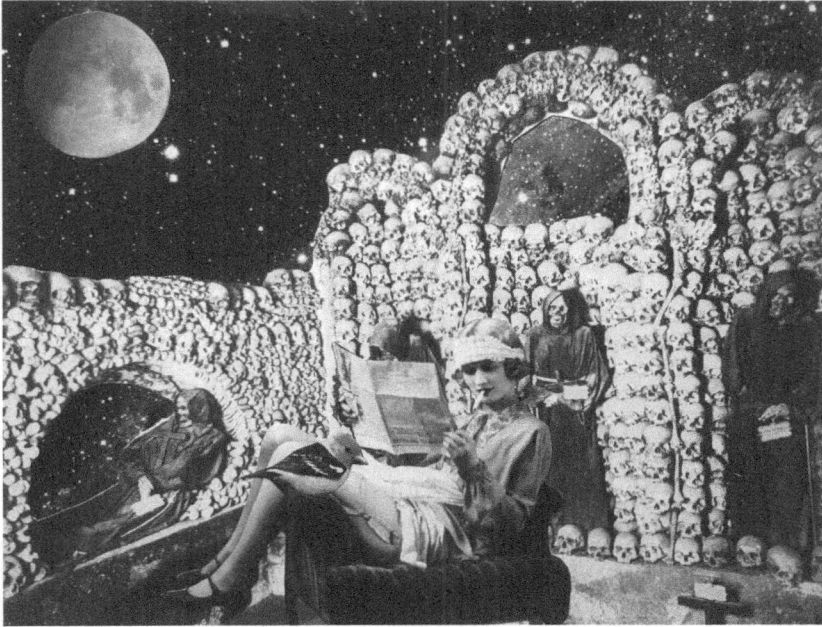

Figure 3: Previous Coping

PURPOSE

Coping strategies are actions a person may take to provide relief and resolution during challenging times (Worden, 2018). A person's coping strategy in previous losses will impact and inform the course of their current grieving and may be classified in a variety of ways.

Worden (2018) provided three types of coping strategies: problem-solving, active emotional, and avoidant emotional. The problem-solving coping style is used to describe how an individual uses systematic strategies to address the challenges that may occur due to loss. Those who engage in active emotional coping style express their true feelings, reframe their experiences to emphasize their positive aspects, and accept support from others. Those with an avoidant emotional style engage in activities that may be detrimental, such as social withdrawal, distraction, blaming others, and denial, instead of directly addressing their problems.

Of these three strategies, clearly those who engage in avoidant emotional strategies face the greatest risk of experiencing complicated grief (Worden, 2018). Identifying and understanding a client's past coping strategies can aid in planning for future grief counseling, helping the therapist be aware of potential pitfalls that may exist and build upon previous strengths. For example, if a client expresses that when feeling stress or grief, they rely on various substances to avoid feeling pain, the therapist can implement and provide healthy stress-management strategies and positive coping skills. Contrarily, if a client expresses that they were previously successful in overcoming their challenges through the help of support groups, the therapist can help the client identify and locate similar resources.

GOAL

The process may address all four Tasks of Mourning, helping the client explore ways they have previously addressed loss and grief and what current strategies they may be using. It allows for goal formation related to healthy coping mechanisms and their implementation.

MATERIALS

Paper or canvas	Crayons
Paint	Magazine/book clippings
Markers/pens	Scissors
Color pencils	Glue
Pastels	Clay/Model Magic

INSTRUCTION

Ask the client to consider previous times they experienced loss and grief, and how they had coped with them. What strategies did they use to work through their loss? What did their coping look like?

When they are ready, ask them to create a piece representing their previous coping strategies.

POSSIBLE PROCESSING QUESTIONS AND PROMPTS

After your client completes their piece, ask them to take time and reflect on their creation and consider their previous coping strategies. The following questions may be used to further explore the process.

1. Can you tell me about your creation and how it represents your previous coping strategies?

2. How would you describe your previous coping strategies? What did these strategies look like?

3. How do you think these strategies were helpful? Unhelpful?

4. Which of these previous strategies do you use in your current grief journey?

5. Do you think your current coping strategies are helpful? If so, which ones? How are they helpful?

6. Are there any coping strategies that you feel are harmful to you? Which ones? How are they harmful?

7. Are there strategies you could add that would be beneficial to you? What would this look like?

8. Are there any changes you would like to see in how you currently cope compared to previous coping? How could you create these changes?

BLOCKS

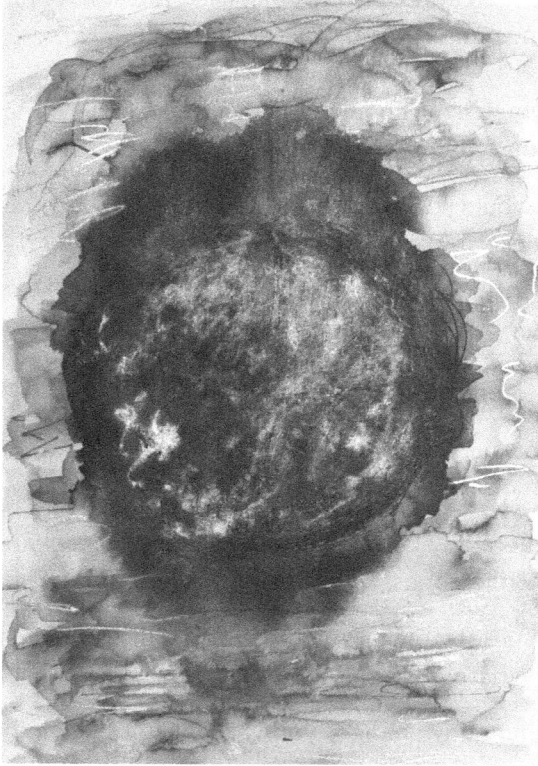

Figure 4: Blocks

PURPOSE

When a person seeks therapy to help them work through their grief, it may be assumed that they are ready for and committed to the process. There are times when such assumptions are erroneous. It is possible that while they may be aware of their need for help, they may also feel that they cannot fully commit to the act of grieving (Worden, 2018).

The reasons for this resistance may vary greatly. Self-blocking could be a sign that a client is not ready to accept the reality of their loss (Worden, 2018). It could also indicate that a client is fearful or wishes to avoid any challenging emotional responses they may experience. The client may not even be aware they are engaged in such blocking.

However, in other cases, the client may be aware of their blocking behaviors, but feel justified in doing so. They may tell themselves that their reason for such avoidance is a matter of survival or self-protection. For example, one client who lost her husband explained that she could not participate in grief counseling because she was unwilling to accept that her husband was truly gone; it was simply too much for her to bear. She believed that she was unable to withstand the emotional toll of accepting his death, and by doing so would cause irreparable damage. She was unwilling to take the risk.

Examining the blocks a person has created allows for reality testing and the challenging of thought distortions that may be preventing effective grieving. When a person chooses not to fully engage with their grieving process, they create increased risks for more difficult grief and in some cases greater risks of complicated grief.

GOAL

This directive addresses the 1st and 2nd Task of Mourning. It focuses on exploring blocks the client may have that prevent them from fully engaging with their grief. By promoting reflection of their fears and any thought distortions, it allows for goal formation around actions that can be taken to overcome these blockages.

MATERIALS

Paper or canvas	Crayons
Paint	Magazine/book clippings
Markers/pens	Scissors
Color pencils	Glue
Pastels	Clay/Model Magic

INSTRUCTION

Ask the client to take a few moments to consider their grief journey so far. Where do they feel they have made progress? Where are they feeling stuck? When they are ready, ask them to create a piece depicting any blockages they feel are preventing them from fully grieving.

POSSIBLE PROCESSING QUESTIONS AND PROMPTS

After your client completes their piece, ask them to take time to reflect on what they have created. The following questions may be used to further explore the process.

1. Can you tell me about the piece you created?

2. Can you explain how your piece shows your progress? Your blocks?

3. Why do you feel you are blocked in the areas you identified?

4. Do these blocks come from inside you or are they external?

5. Do you feel the blocks to your grief serve a purpose? If so, what is this purpose?

6. How are these blockages impacting you and your grief?

7. How do you feel when you consider removing these barriers? What do you feel emotionally? Physically?

8. If you had to choose one word to describe your feelings about moving beyond your blocks and grieving fully, what would that word be? What does this word mean to you?

9. When you consider removing the blocks and fully engaging in grieving, how do you feel emotionally? Physically?

10. What steps do you think you could take to break down these barriers to grief? How would that feel? How would it change the way you view and experience your grief?

PERMISSION TO GRIEVE

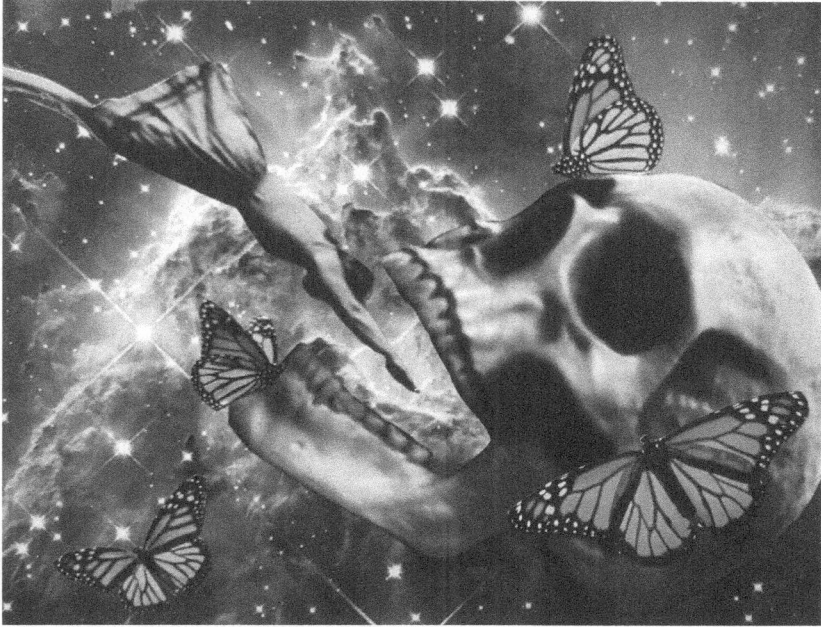

Figure 5: Permission to Grieve

PURPOSE

For some, grief can feel overwhelming, filled with conflicting and confusing emotions and uncomfortable physical symptoms (Lobb et al., 2010). The bereaved may not only experience difficult emotions such as anger, despair, longing, and fear, but pain and exhaustion as well (Worden, 2018). This can be especially true when someone is experiencing disenfranchised grief, as they may begin to view their grief as hidden, inappropriate, or invalid (Doka, 2002).

These beliefs do not change the experience of grief but may create more obstacles by invalidating their own feelings and experiences. When a person prevents themselves from effectively grieving, they increase their risk of developing complicated grief (Shear, 2012).

To effectively grieve, there may be times where a person needs to consciously validate their own feelings and give themselves permission to grieve (Worden, 2018). This is especially true for those experiencing disenfranchised grief, as they do not have the same social support as others (Doka, 2002).

By giving themselves permission to fully grieve, they may become more empathetic and accepting of their own needs. They may begin to view their emotional and physical reactions as valid and worthy of attention and acceptance. Permission may increase feelings of self-efficacy, self-acceptance, and hope.

GOAL

This process addresses the 1st and 2nd Task of Mourning. It focuses on helping someone examine and challenge their core beliefs about the appropriateness of their grief, and instills validity of their feelings, and acceptance of their grief journey. It facilitates self-acceptance, self-efficacy, and mastery.

MATERIALS

Paper or canvas	Crayons
Paint	Magazine/book clippings
Markers/pens	Scissors
Color pencils	Glue
Pastels	Clay/Model Magic

INSTRUCTION

Ask the client to reflect on their feelings related to the validity of their grief and its associated emotions. Do they feel they are accepting of their grief and its needs? Do they feel they have the right to grieve? Ask them to consider what it means to give themselves permission to grieve. Have they given themselves this permission? When they are ready, ask them to create a piece around what it means to give themselves permission to grieve.

POSSIBLE PROCESSING QUESTIONS AND PROMPTS

After your client completes their piece, ask them to take time to consider their creation and the feelings expressed within it. The following questions may be used to further explore the process.

1. Can you tell me about your creation? What elements stick out to you? Why?

2. What does the idea of permission mean to you?

3. Do you feel like your grief is seen and heard? How or how not? Has this changed the way you feel about your grief?

4. What does it mean to validate your own feelings? To be validated by others?

5. Have you noticed a change in the way others respond to your grief from the initial loss to now? If so, what does that change look like? How has this change impacted you?

6. Have you noticed any changes in your behaviors due to your grief either being recognized or not? If so, what has changed?

7. How do you feel about being given permission to grieve? What if the permission came from an outside source? What if that permission came from you?

8. How do you think having permission to grieve would change how you feel about your grief? How you process it?

9. What do you think you need to give yourself this permission? What steps can you take to give yourself this permission?

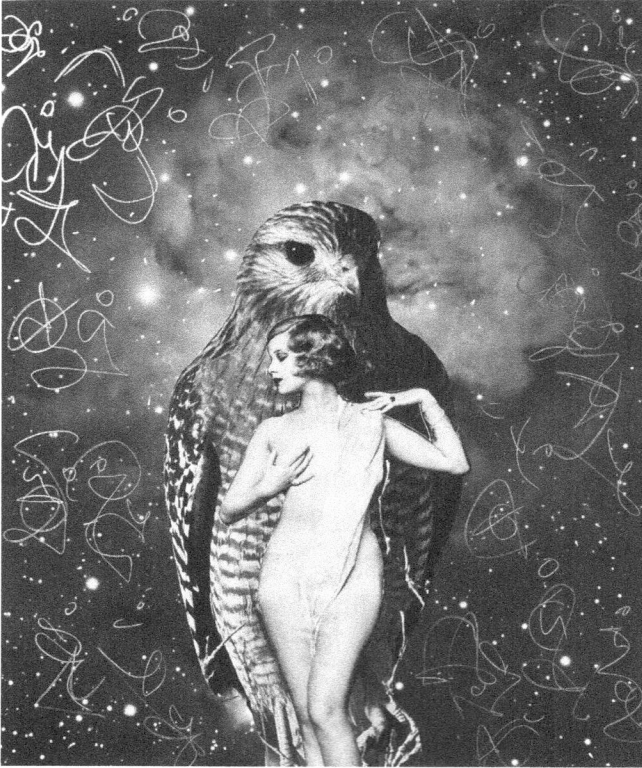

Figure 6: Safety

PURPOSE

Loss can have dramatic and long-term effects on someone (Worden, 2018). The person may feel that their whole life has been turned upside down and the world has changed in ways that may seem more threatening. Safety and security may be shattered, feelings that are magnified if the loss was sudden or unexpected. Their sense of what good health means, something up until then may have been taken for granted, is challenged. They may even feel unsafe in the world around them.

When such a client feels unsafe, they may begin to block their own grief (Worden, 2018). They may engage in avoiding behaviors that impact their ability to function. They may experience increased fear and anxiety that, when left unaddressed, may become debilitating and place them at increased risk for complicated grief.

Often, therapists set a goal to create a safe space for the client to explore themselves and their current concerns (Worden, 2018). In grief and trauma, feelings of emotional safety need to be extended beyond the confines of the therapist's office and into the person's daily experiences to facilitate progress and functioning. Examining what the client needs to feel safe again is the first significant step (Sieff, 2015).

GOAL

This directive addresses the 2nd Task of Mourning. The focus is to help the client explore the idea of safety, how safe they currently feel, and what they need to feel secure again. It further allows for creating goals to help the client reach a self-identified safe space and increase feelings of self-efficacy and hope.

MATERIALS

Paper or canvas	Crayons
Paint	Magazine/book clippings
Markers/pens	Scissors
Color pencils	Glue
Pastels	Clay/Model Magic

INSTRUCTION

Ask the client to take a few moments to consider the idea of safety. What is safety? What does it mean to feel safe? What makes them feel safe? Ask them to consider their current feelings of safety. When they are ready, ask them to create a piece around their idea of safety.

POSSIBLE PROCESSING QUESTIONS AND PROMPTS

After your client completes their piece, ask them to take time to consider the what they have created. The following questions may be used to further explore the process.

1. Can you tell me about your piece and how it reflects your idea of safety?

2. What does it mean to be "safe"?

3. How safe do you feel currently? How has this changed since your loss?

4. What element of your loss has made you feel unsafe?

5. In general, what makes you feel safe? Unsafe? Why?

6. How do you think your behaviors change when you feel safe versus when you feel unsafe?

7. How do you think your emotions change when you feel safe versus unsafe?

8. How do you think feeling safer would impact your grief? Your life in general?

9. How much control do you feel you have over your feelings of safety?

10. What would help you to feel safer?

11. Are there any actions you could take that would help you increase your feelings of safety? What are they?

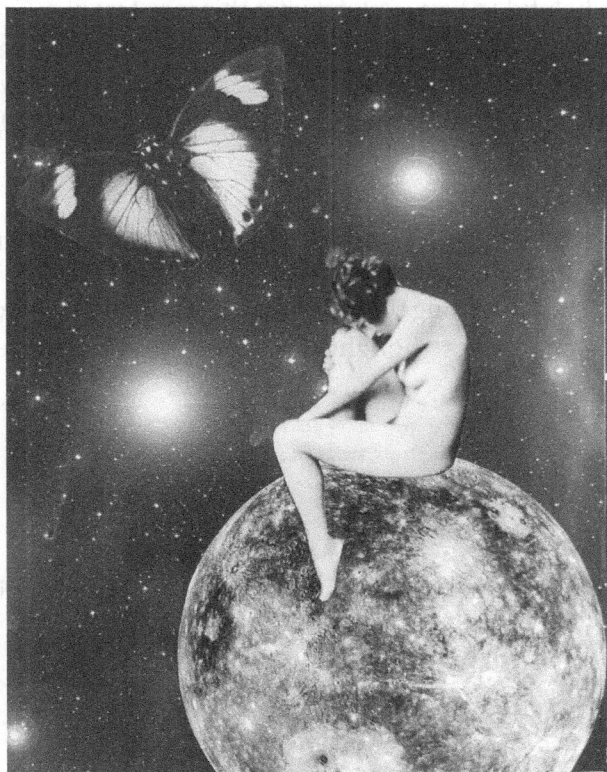

Figure 7: Sitting with Sorrow

PURPOSE

A person may resist fully embracing their feelings when confronted with the often intense emotional responses to grief (Worden, 2018). While some do engage with the experience and confront the feeling, others may avoid such pain. I would argue that one of the most difficult things a person can do in therapy is to sit with their difficult emotions and hold space for their own pain and suffering without engaging in avoidant thoughts or behaviors (Worden, 2018). It is not uncommon for the bereaved to push away their feelings of sorrow, until they become so overwhelmed by the emotion it becomes all-consuming, impacting daily functioning (Mason et al., 2020). Such avoidance places a person at an increased risk of complicated grief by interrupting the healthy—and necessary—emotional reactions.

Since fully experiencing painful emotions is likely overwhelming, it may be helpful to first explore what this may feel like. Creating an opportunity for a person to visualize and contemplate the experience before allowing themselves to feel the emotion may stave off any thought distortions and—in turn—increase feelings of self-efficacy.

GOAL

This directive addresses the 2nd Task of Mourning. It expects the client to consider their emotions and how it might feel to "be" with them instead of avoiding them. It promotes mindfulness techniques. It further challenges thought distortions and facilitates reality testing.

MATERIALS

Paper or canvas	Crayons
Paint	Magazine/book clippings
Markers/pens	Scissors
Color pencils	Glue
Pastels	Clay/Model Magic

INSTRUCTION

Ask the client to consider their distressing grief emotions and their reactions to them. How do they react when they begin to feel these emotions? What actions do they take in response to their emotions? When they are ready, ask them to create a piece that reflects how they feel or would feel about sitting with their sorrow.

POSSIBLE PROCESSING QUESTIONS AND PROMPTS

After your client completes their piece, ask them to reflect on their creation. The following questions may be used to further explore the process.

1. Can you tell me about this piece? How do you think it represents your reaction to feeling the painful emotions of grief?

2. When you begin to feel difficult emotions how do you react? What thoughts do you have? What actions do you take?

3. How did it feel to consider sitting with your feelings? Did you notice any changes in your body? What thoughts were your having?

4. How did you feel creating this piece? Did you notice any changes in your body? Emotions?

5. How do you think holding space for your emotions would impact you? Your grief?

6. How comfortable are you with sitting with these feelings and giving them the space to just be? What would make you more comfortable? Less comfortable?

7. How could you change your previous thoughts and feelings about experiencing the emotions of grief? How do you think changing your thoughts might change your reaction to your feelings? How do you think these changes would impact your grief?

8. What steps do you think you could take to begin to allow yourself to sit with your sorrow?

ANGER

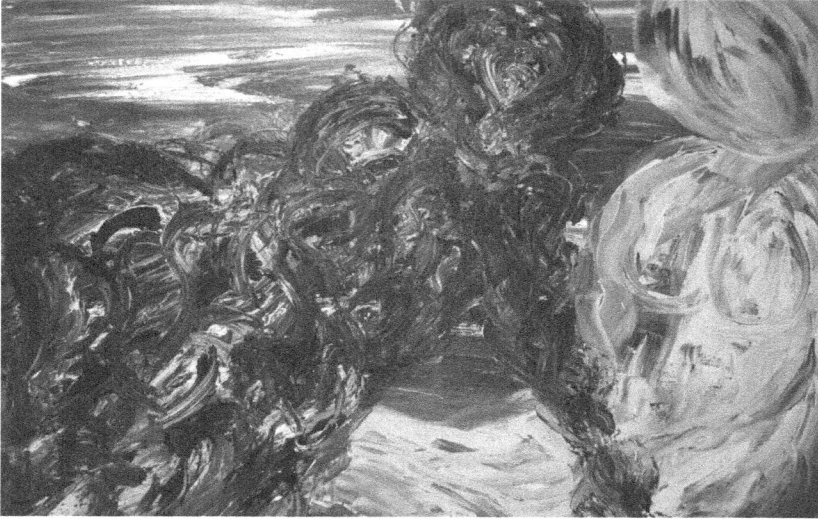

Figure 8: Anger

PURPOSE

Grief causes many emotions for the bereaved (Worden, 2018), including anger, one of the most common and at times most difficult to address. As loss is often outside of a person's control, the bereaved may feel frustrated and helpless, primary emotions that when not addressed immediately can become anger (Beck & Beck, 2011). In a victim of trauma, the anger may be turned towards their perpetrator or, often, themselves (Novaco & Chemtob, 1998).

Anger is not only limited to one aspect of the loss. For example, a woman may feel angry that her husband has died suddenly while feeling angry of societal expectations that she continues with her life. To complicate matters even further, there may be additional anger if the relationship with the deceased was one of conflict.

When anger isn't expressed and processed, it can be directed towards those around the bereaved, or inward upon themselves

(Silove et al., 2017). They may begin to lash out at others at work or home, causing further damage to those relationships, resulting in alienation and further losses. Unprocessed anger is not only a risk factor for developing complicated grief (Shear, 2015), but may also be a symptom of post-traumatic stress disorder, further compounding the complications (Novaco & Chemtob, 1998).

A person's resultant anger may be so complex that more intensive therapy is required (Novaco & Chemtob, 1998). However, recognizing that the anger is a natural part of the grieving process normalizes it and may help defuse it, and following with further exploration and reflection through art may help (Thompson & Neimeyer, 2014).

GOAL

This process addresses the 2nd Task of Mourning. The focus is to validate and normalize the client's anger and help them begin to process it in a way that minimizes potential harm. It also facilitates potential goals that deal with emotion regulation and behavior modification.

MATERIALS

Paper or canvas	Crayons
Paint	Magazine/book clippings
Markers/pens	Scissors
Color pencils	Glue
Pastels	Clay/Model Magic

INSTRUCTION

Ask the client to take consider any anger they may be experiencing related to their loss. What is causing them to feel angry? Do they feel this anger is impacting their lives? When they are ready, ask them to create a piece that shows their feelings of anger and its impact on them.

POSSIBLE PROCESSING QUESTIONS AND PROMPTS

After your client completes their piece, ask them to take time to consider what they have created. The following questions may be used to further explore the process.

1. Can you tell me about this piece and what elements of anger it shows?

2. If your piece could talk, what would it say?

3. How did it feel to think about your anger? To create a piece around your anger?

4. How have you expressed your anger before now? What actions have you taken when angry?

5. What are your thoughts on how your anger has been expressed? Was this expression helpful? Harmful? How?

6. Do you think your anger has impacted your grieving? How?

7. Do you notice any changes in how you were feeling before creating this piece and after? What changed?

8. What do you think your anger needs? What steps could you take to meet these needs?

9. How do you think you can use this anger for personal change? What lessons do you think your anger could teach you?

10. Do you feel your anger is having a negative impact on your life? The lives around you? If so, what changes could be made to prevent this negative impact?

GUILT

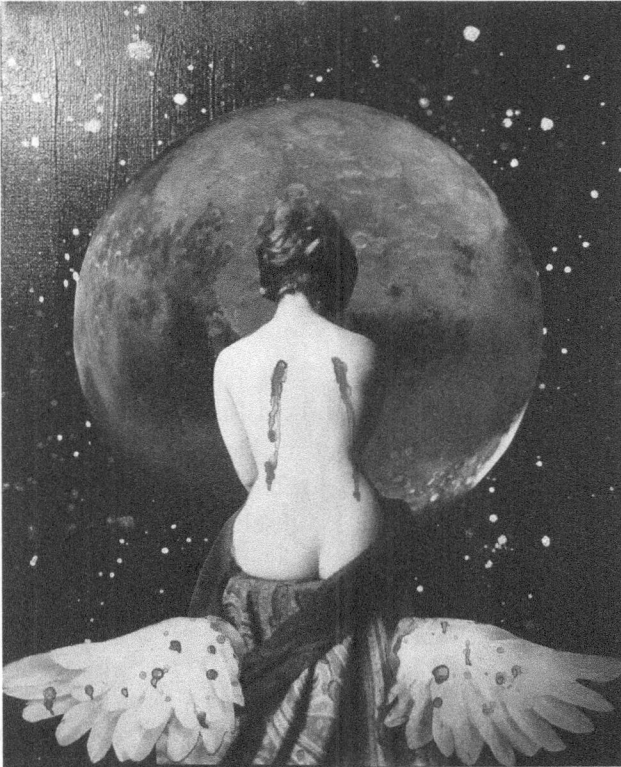

Figure 9: Guilt

PURPOSE

Guilt and self-blame are common reactions to loss and grief (Worden, 2018). The bereaved may believe that they did not do enough to prevent the loss; for example, one client believed if they had taken their mother to the doctor sooner, she would not have died from cancer. Others may feel that they were directly responsible for their loss. One woman blamed her sexual assault on her "foolish" decision to walk down an empty street alone at night.

Such reactions resulting in guilt are irrational (Worden, 2018).

Reality testing and cognitive behavioral therapy can assist in helping the client realize this and allow them to accept that they in fact were not responsible. They may then be able to accept what they were responsible for, process the emotion, and reintegrate it into their overall grief journey.

Still, there are others who experience guilt for actual responsibilities leading to the loss they have experienced (Rando, 1984); for example, a woman who was drinking and driving and caused an accident that resulted in the death of a passenger and her own disability. Another woman may grieve losing her children who were removed by the courts because of her criminal behavior. Even in these cases, where the guilt may be rational and well placed, it still requires exploration and processing to facilitate a healthy journey with grief.

GOAL

This process addresses the 2nd and 3rd Task of Mourning. The focus is to examine and evaluate the realistic basis of the guilt related to the client's loss. This further allows for creating goals that are directed at improving self-talk strategies and self-forgiveness.

MATERIALS

Paper or canvas	Crayons
Paint	Magazine/book clippings
Markers/pens	Scissors
Color pencils	Glue
Pastels	Clay/Model Magic

INSTRUCTION

Ask the client to consider any feelings of guilt they may be experiencing. Ask that they try to view their source of guilt more objectively, perhaps as something separate from them. What does this guilt look and feel like? When they are ready, ask them to create a piece around their feelings of guilt and its impact on them and their grief.

POSSIBLE PROCESSING QUESTIONS AND PROMPTS

After your client completes their piece, ask them to take time to observe their creation. The following questions may be used to further explore the process.

1. Can you tell me about your piece? What feelings did you have while creating it? What feelings do you have looking at it now?

2. How does your art express your feelings of guilt?

3. What do you feel is the source of your guilt?

4. How did it feel to reflect on guilt? Did you notice any emotional changes? Did you notice any changes in your body?

5. When you look at your feelings of guilt, do you think the guilt is accurate? How or how not?

6. How do you think feelings of guilt have impacted your grieving process?

7. How have your feelings of guilt changed the way you talk to yourself? Your self-esteem?

8. How do you think your self-talk impacts your daily functioning? Your ability to grieve?

9. Are there any changes you would like to make regarding your feelings of guilt? What steps could your take to help you create these changes?

FEAR

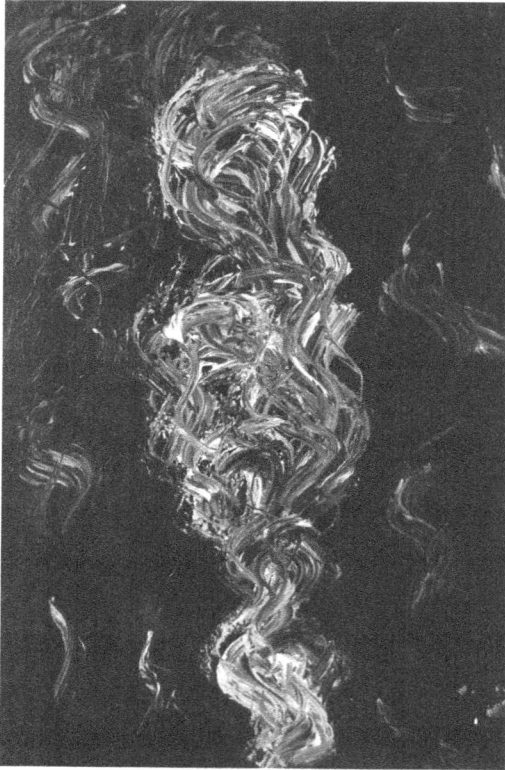

Figure 10: Fear

PURPOSE

Fear is common, a dynamic element of grief (Rando, 1984) and may be experienced and expressed in various ways depending on the client and their loss. A client may fear for their own health and safety or for their living loved ones, and that others they love may die as well. If loss is due to a divorce, a client may be frightened of their new status as a single person. Those who have turned to drugs and alcohol as a way to escape a loss or mute their grieving may eventually become frightened about their inability to function in the world without their substance of choice.

Such fear, when left unacknowledged, often impacts a person's ability to function and may lead to helplessness and hopelessness, further creating a barrier to effective grief processing, potentially leading to complicated grief (Worden, 2018). It may also cause the client to take actions to avoid their feared outcome. For example, they may shun from creating new relationships or end current ones to avoid the anticipated pain of potentially losing someone else.

By exploring such fear, the client is provided an opportunity to challenge the potentially resultant irrational thoughts (Worden, 2018). This may begin to help the client regain feelings of self-efficacy and hope, allowing for the facilitation of positive emotional and behavioral change.

GOAL

This process addresses the 2nd and 3rd Task of Mourning. The focus is to help the client explore any fear they may be experiencing because of their loss. It allows the client to examine how this fear may be impacting their actions and their grief. It further allows for challenging their fear-based thought distortions and creating strategies to improve identified avoidant behaviors.

MATERIALS

Paper or canvas	Crayons
Paint	Magazine/book clippings
Markers/pens	Scissors
Color pencils	Glue
Pastels	Clay/Model Magic

INSTRUCTION

Ask the client to take a few moments to reflect on any fear they may be experiencing. What are they afraid of? What does their fear look like? What does it feel like? When they are ready, ask them to create a piece that depicts their fear.

POSSIBLE PROCESSING QUESTIONS AND PROMPTS

After your client completes their piece, ask them to take time to consider what they have created. The following questions may be used to further explore the process.

1. Can you tell me about your piece? How does it represent your fear?

2. How did it feel to consider and face this fear through your creation?

3. Did you notice any changes in your emotions or body as you were creating your piece? If so, what changed?

4. When you are feeling fearful, what happens to your thoughts? Your actions? How do you feel it in your body?

5. Do you feel your fear is impacting your life? Your grief? How so?

6. If your piece could talk, what do you think it would say?

7. What do you think your fear needs? How can you meet those needs?

8. Do you feel like the fear you identified in your piece is helping or hurting you? How so?

9. What makes you feel as though your fear is valid? Invalid?

10. Are there any changes you would like to see related to your fear? If so, what would those changes look like? What steps could you take to create these changes?

ANXIETY

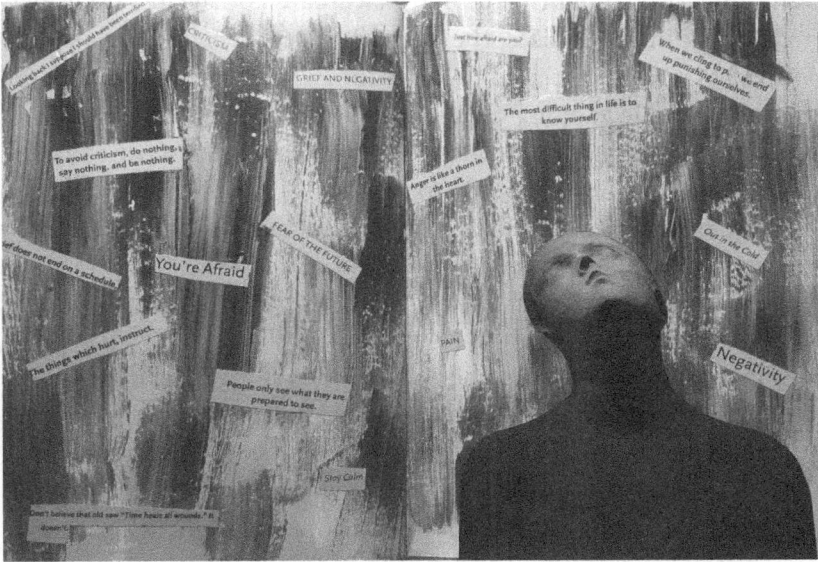

Figure 11: Anxiety

PURPOSE

Those who grieve often feel anxiety as they begin to experience increased fears and pressures of the unknown after their loss (Worden, 2018). They must make sudden and sometimes drastic life changes for which they may feel unprepared. For example, a man's young wife dies leaving him to care for their two small children. In addition to grieving his wife, the widower must also adjust to a new life where he is a single father and solely responsible for the wellbeing of his children. As the man struggles to adjust to his new reality, anxiety of the unexpected and the unknown may emerge.

Grief-related anxiety can range in intensity depending on the type of loss and extent of ensuing life changes. For some, anxiety may manifest as low levels of insecurity, while for others it may emerge as debilitating panic attacks. Physical symptoms, including racing heart, difficulty sleeping, and trouble eating, may begin to impact daily living. More extreme levels of anxiety may indicate a burgeoning anxiety disorder, requiring further assessment and more intensive intervention.

To complicate matters, it is possible for a person to have a preexisting anxiety disorder that is then exacerbated by the loss (Marques et al., 2013). In these cases, the client may report increased anxiety symptoms and heightened debilitation. These clients are at even greater risk of developing complicated grief.

By being made aware of and confronting the potential cause and rationale of the emergent anxiety, a client can begin to identify techniques that may help stave off the debilitating symptoms. It may also increase empowerment and control.

GOAL

This process addresses the 2nd Task of Mourning. The objective is to help the client explore the underlying anxiety they may be experiencing and uncover its source and needs. It challenges any thought distortions and promotes reality testing to help develop goals that focus on eradicating maladaptive behaviors and identifying potentially beneficial grounding and mindfulness techniques.

MATERIALS

Paper or canvas	Crayons
Paint	Magazine/book clippings
Markers/pens	Scissors
Color pencils	Glue
Pastels	Clay/Model Magic

INSTRUCTION

Ask the client to take a few moments to consider any anxiety they may be currently experiencing. What does this anxiety look like? How does it impact them? What does this anxiety feel like emotionally and physically? When they are ready, ask them to create a piece related to their anxiety and its impact on them and their grief.

POSSIBLE PROCESSING QUESTIONS AND PROMPTS

After your client completes their piece, ask them to take time to consider what they have created. The following questions may be used to further explore the process.

1. Can you describe your piece and how it reflects your anxiety?

2. If your piece could talk, what do you think it would say?

3. Have you noticed any triggers to your anxious feelings?

4. When you are feeling anxious, how does this impact your feelings? Your body sensations? Your actions?

5. How did it feel to consider and face this anxiety through your creation?

6. Did you notice any changes in your emotions or body as you were creating your piece? If so, what changed?

7. Do you feel your anxiety is impacting your life? Your grief? How so?

8. What do you think would help you feel less anxious?

9. Are there any techniques you have tried previously when you have experienced anxiety? What were they? What was their impact on your anxiety and your functioning?

10. Are there any changes you would like to see related to your anxiety? If so, what would those changes look like? What steps could you take to create these changes?

CONFLICTING EMOTIONS

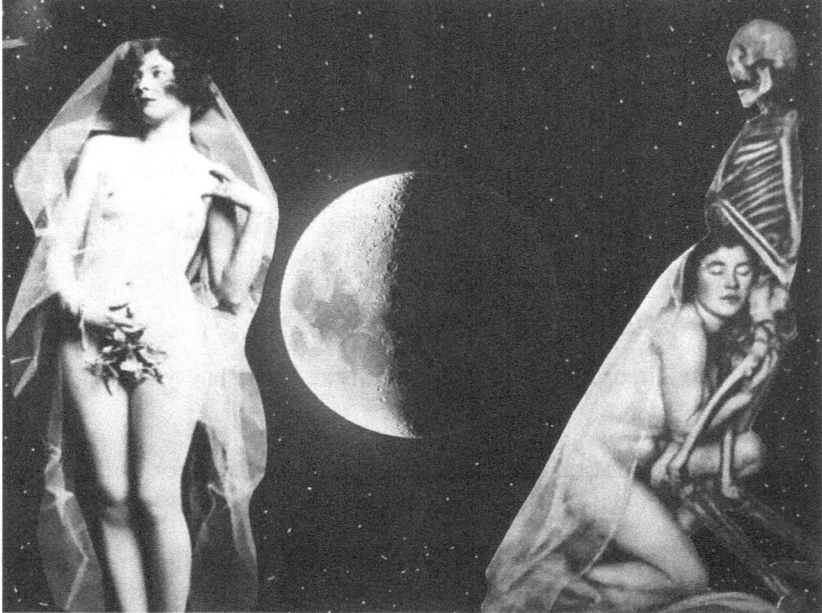

Figure 12: Conflicting Emotions

PURPOSE

Loss can result in a wide range of emotional reactions, including sadness, blame, shock, yearning, emancipation, relief, and numbness (Worden, 2018). At times these emotions may conflict with one another. For example, if an elderly parent dies after years of dementia, their adult children may feel sadness but also relief, maybe even joy. Or a woman who has received a mastectomy may feel relieved that she has mitigated her breast cancer and potentially reduced her future risks but also feel regret and sadness for the loss.

Such conflicting emotions may create additional distress (Worden, 2018). They may feel that they cannot express such inner emotional turmoil because others may not understand or accept them. They may even question or doubt their own justifications for feeling so.

Those prone to rigid, either/or thought processes may express greater confusion and discomfort, unable to accept that they can or are allowed to experience and express such seemingly disparate emotions. When such a client believes their emotions conflict with social norms, such as feeling relief or even joy when someone dies, they may disenfranchise their own grief (Doka, 2002), sometimes resulting in shame or guilt. This may cause further, more embedded, distress and impede the necessary grieving processes.

In instances of such conflicting emotions, it may be beneficial for the therapist to explore and validate all emotional reactions of the client and potential strategies to reduce perceived conflict (Bonanno, 2001). Such validation and eventual integration may foster personal acceptance and alleviate feelings of confusion or additional distress.

GOAL

This process addresses the 2nd Task of Mourning. The objective is to help the client explore conflicting emotions, and further acknowledge, validate, and process them, eventually helping them develop goals that focus on integrating these seemingly conflicting emotions.

MATERIALS

Paper or canvas	Crayons
Paint	Magazine/book clippings
Markers/pens	Scissors
Color pencils	Glue
Pastels	Clay/Model Magic

INSTRUCTION

Ask the client to take a few moments to consider any emotions they are experiencing that they feel conflict with each other. What emotions are do they feel are opposite and incompatible with each other? When they are ready, ask them to create a piece that represents their conflicting emotions and their impact on their grieving and lives in general.

POSSIBLE PROCESSING QUESTIONS AND PROMPTS

After your client completes their piece, ask them to take time to reflect on what they have created. The following questions may be used to further explore the process.

1. Can you tell me about your creation? What emotions did you identify as being in conflict?

2. Why do you feel these emotions are incompatible?

3. How does the feeling of conflict impact you and your grief?

4. Do you think both emotions are fully valid? Partly valid? Invalid? How so?

5. Do you feel you can experience both emotions as equal and valid? Why or why not?

6. What would help you reconcile these emotions, giving them both the care and attention they need?

7. How do you think this would impact your grief moving forward?

8. What do you think the first emotion is trying to tell you? What does it need?

9. What do you think the second emotion is trying to tell you? What does it need?

10. What steps can you take to help meet the needs of both emotions? How do you think meeting these needs will change your grief?

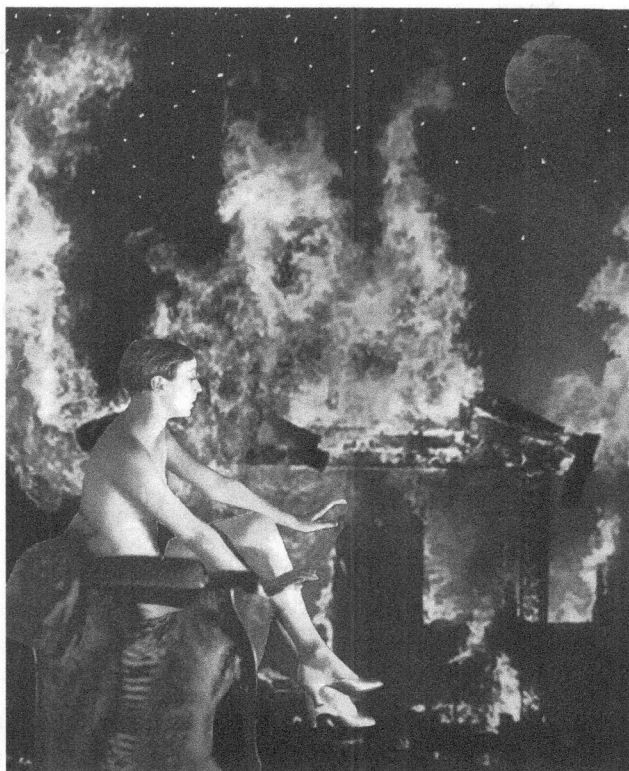

Figure 13: Intrusive Thoughts

PURPOSE

Intrusive thoughts are images or ideas that occur without control or warning and tend to be disturbing in nature (Boelen & Huntjens, 2008). While intrusive thoughts are not unique to grief, they tend to take a particular form when the grief is related to a death. In death-related losses, a person may mentally replay their memories of the death or what they imagine about it. If the client was present when their loved one dies, they may experience intense memories that often focus on perceived suffering or pain.

Ironically, these thoughts may become particularly gruesome and distressing if the client was not present at the death but is aware that the death was violent, such as a murder or suicide. In such cases, an individual may attempt to recreate or imagine the final moments for the victim, often focusing on how painful the situation was or how much they suffered.

In non-death-related losses, intrusive thoughts may include reliving a particular trauma, imagining how much worse it could have been (Worden, 2018). Such thoughts can feel constant, with no end in sight, particularly soon after the loss or trauma. These thoughts may cause increased distress, difficulty sleeping, and result in disruption of daily living.

Regardless of what caused the intrusive thought or what such thoughts consist of, it can be quite distressing, often appearing suddenly and without warning. They may begin to impede grief by causing a client to avoid situations where they are reminded of their loss, potentially triggering an intrusive thought (Worden, 2018).

GOAL

This process addresses the 2nd Task of Mourning. Its objective is to help the client examine intrusive thoughts they may have related to their loss. It provides opportunities to validate the distress these thoughts cause while helping them create goals that may help mitigate their impact on a person's functioning. By exploring the intrusive thought, its triggers, and emotional and behavioral impacts, a client can begin to decrease their feelings of distress and increase feelings of self-efficacy.

MATERIALS

Paper or canvas	Crayons
Paint	Magazine/book clippings
Markers/pens	Scissors
Color pencils	Glue
Pastels	Clay/Model Magic

INSTRUCTION

Ask the client to take a few moments to reflect on any intrusive thoughts they may be experiencing related to their loss. How are these thoughts impacting their functioning? What emotions are the thoughts causing in them? How are these thoughts impacting their behaviors? When they are ready, ask that they create a piece related to their recurring intrusive thoughts.

POSSIBLE PROCESSING QUESTIONS AND PROMPTS

After your client completes their piece, ask them to take time to reflect on what they have created. The following questions may be used to further explore the process.

1. Can you tell me a bit about your intrusive thoughts and the piece you have created?

2. If you had to assign one word to these thoughts and the art you created, what would it be? What does this word mean to you?

3. When you reflect on these thoughts do you see any patterns or triggers?

4. Do you feel these thoughts and the scenarios they recreate are accurate? How or how not?

5. Is there anything that seems to make these thoughts better? Worse?

6. What changes do you notice in your body when these thoughts occur? In your behavior?

7. What do you think would help relieve the distress of these thoughts?

8. What actions do you think you could take when the intrusive thoughts begin to regain control of your thoughts/actions?

MEMORY

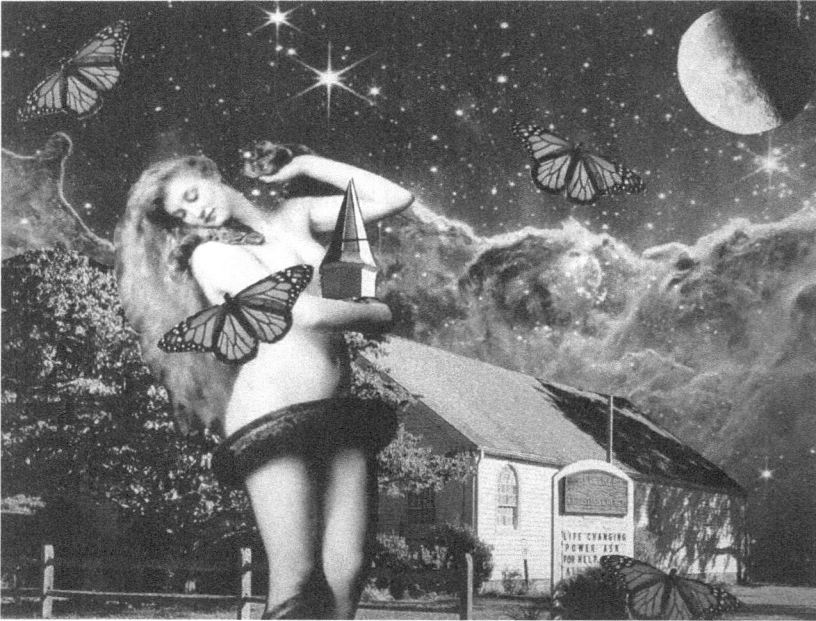

Figure 14: Memory

PURPOSE

After experiencing a loss, all that may remain may be the memories of what or who was lost. Therapists often encourage "reminiscing" or engaging in a "life review" (i.e., sharing memories of the deceased) (Worden, 2018, p.240). This allows those who are grieving to feel greater connection with what or whom they lost, and potentially create and develop more positive emotions, perhaps even joy in such remembrance. It may further result in expanded social support as they share their memories with another. This has been found particularly beneficial for the elderly.

Of course, not all memories are positive; yet sharing negative or challenging memories may also provide an opportunity to process them, perhaps leading to further validation. This may allow an opportunity for clients to explore their memories as a more complete, holistic experience.

Life review may often become particularly important for those experiencing disenfranchised grief (Doka, 2002). Since disenfranchised grief is not seen or validated by society, the bereaved may not have the opportunity to share their memories with others. For example, a woman who had a long-term intimate relationship with a married man who suddenly died may feel that she cannot share her grief over his passing or her memories of their relationship due to the secret nature of the affair. Yet, the loss is not diminished because the relationship was not publicly acknowledged, it is just more secretive. The ability to share these memories within a safe therapeutic relationship may promote effective processing of such grief and further prevent complicated grief.

GOAL

This process may address all four Tasks of Mourning. It provides the client an opportunity to share their memories of their loved ones and explore how the relationship impacted their lives. This reinforces meaning making, and provides an opportunity for emotional processing, reintegration, and reality testing. It further facilitates goal formation.

MATERIALS

Paper or canvas	Crayons
Paint	Magazine/book clippings
Markers/pens	Scissors
Color pencils	Glue
Pastels	Clay/Model Magic

INSTRUCTION

Ask the client to take a few moments to remember the person who has passed and a memory they have of this person. Where were they?

What were they doing? When they have had time to reflect ask them to create an image of this memory using the materials provided.

POSSIBLE PROCESSING QUESTIONS AND PROMPTS

After your client completes their piece, ask them to take time to observe their creation and reflect on their selected memory. The following questions may be used to further explore the process.

1. Can you tell me about your piece? How does it depict your memory?

2. Why did you select this memory?

3. How did it feel to share this memory?

4. Is there anything about this memory and the piece you have created that sticks out to you?

5. When you first considered this memory did you notice any changes in your body? If so, what were those changes?

6. How did it feel to create a piece around this memory? Why?

7. How do you think the original experience has impacted you? How does it still impact you?

8. How do you feel the memories of your loved one may impact your future?

9. Are there elements to your memories that you find helpful? Harmful? How so?

10. If there are elements that you find helpful, how could you use this to help you with your grief?

11. If there are elements that you find harmful, how could that harm be reduced in the future?

RELATIONSHIP REALITY

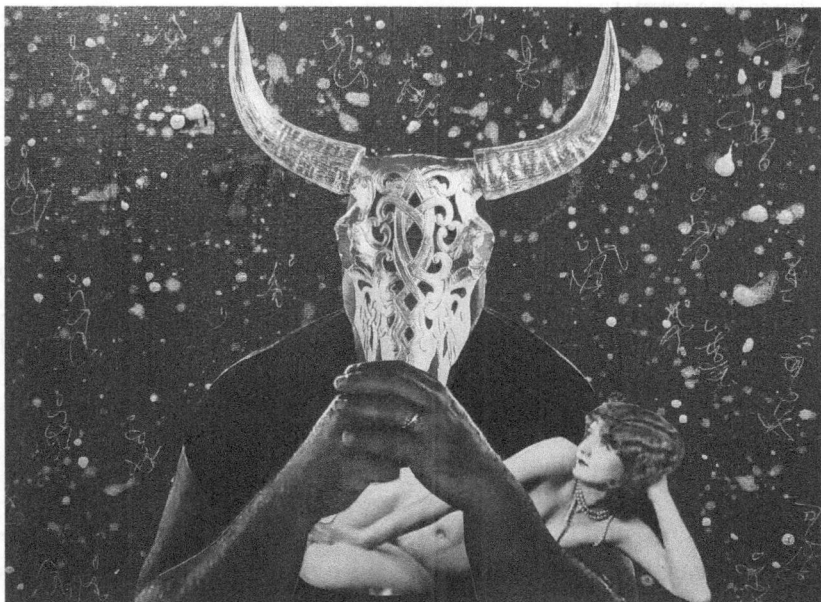

Figure 15: Relationship Reality

PURPOSE

As discussed in the *Memory* directive, reminiscing can have a positive impact in the grief of an individual; but what happens when the relationship was conflicted or abusive? In these cases, the life review may need to be more strategic, carefully considering previous trauma (Figley, 2013).

Those who subscribe to attachment theory recognize that the level of grief a person experiences is directly related to the type of attachment they had for what or who was lost (Bowlby, 2008); thus, the amount of grief or distress a person experiences after the death of someone they were in conflict with is case-specific. Still, the research is not conclusive on the impact that grief has on those who had ambivalent relationships; for some the grief response was minimal and for others the person grieving was at risk of complicated bereavement (Figley, 2013).

In case of the death of an abuser or someone with whom there was a shared conflictual relationship, the relationship may be viewed in terms of extremes, with trauma impacting how they remember those they were in conflict with (Conte, 2002). The person may remember the deceased at times as a warm caregiver, and at other times as a monster.

A woman who did not want to divorce her husband may remember her marriage in glowing terms, either forgetting or refusing to acknowledge the betrayal she felt from her husband's abuse. In other words, she is grieving inaccurate or reprocessed memories of perfection and bliss.

In such scenarios, it is invaluable to help the person experiencing such loss process their grief, helping them recognize relationship needs to be viewed in holistic terms, acknowledging both the positive and negative. This review may challenge thought distortions and aid in more accurate processing of emotions (Worden, 2018).

GOAL

This process potentially addresses all four Tasks of Mourning. It focuses on the potential thought distortions your client may experience regarding their relationship with the deceased. It facilitates emotional processing and expression, critical for reintegration. It promotes goal formation that focuses on identifying their needs.

MATERIALS

Paer or canvas	Crayons
Paint	Magazine/book clippings
Markers/pens	Scissors
Color pencils	Glue
Pastels	Clay/Model Magic

INSTRUCTION

Ask the client to consider their relationship with the deceased. Ask them to consider how the relationship made them feel and how they would describe it to someone else. Ask that they consider all sides of the relationship and reflect on both positive and negative aspects without focusing on only one aspect or taking a judgmental stance. When they are ready, ask them to create an image that represents their relationship as a whole without picking only one part.

POSSIBLE PROCESSING QUESTIONS AND PROMPTS

After your client completes their piece, ask them to consider the image they have created. The following questions may be used to further explore the process.

1. Can you tell me about the piece you have created? How does it represent the many aspects of your relationship?

2. If you had to describe your relationship in one word, what would it be? What does this word mean to you?

3. Do you think this word also accurately describes the art you created? Why or why not?

4. What stands out about the piece you created? Why?

5. How comfortable were you when considering the entire relationship and not just one part or another?

6. Were there any emotions that came up during this reflection that made you uncomfortable? If so, why?

7. How accurately do you think the piece conveys your relationship? Why or why not?

8. Do you feel that considering both the positive and negative aspects of your relationship has changed your overall view of the relationship? If so, how?

9. Are there any emotions that came up that you feel you haven't addressed during your grieving process? If so, what are the emotions? How could they be addressed moving forward?

10. How do you think a more holistic view of your relationship will change your grief?

THINGS LEFT UNSAID

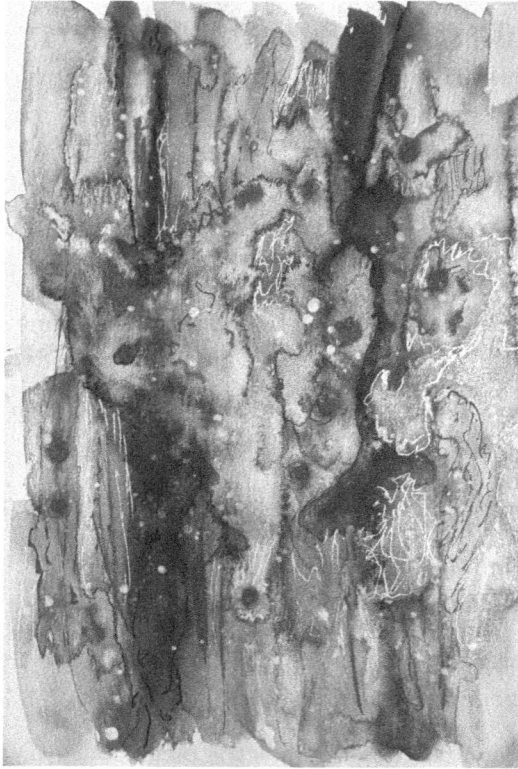

Figure 16: Things Left Unsaid

PURPOSE

Loss is sometimes sudden and unexpected, leaving an individual with "unfinished business," often including issues that were left unaddressed (Worden, 2018). When a death is expected, there is time during the anticipatory grieving process for conversations that were never had to attain closure (Rando, 1984). However, when it is sudden, a person is denied the opportunity for such closure and, in the case of conflictual relationships, to make repairs. This may result in regret or guilt for having been unable to say or do the things they felt they needed (Worden, 2018). As the *Guilt* directive indicates, such unchallenged or processed guilt may further impede effective grieving.

In some cases, a client may feel that they needed an apology or indications of love and affirmation from the deceased before their passing (Worden, 2018). As they learn to accept the loss of the deceased, they must also come to accept that such conversations will never happen. This may result in anger, sorrow, or longing.

While the client cannot have the conversation that they feel they needed, they can explore the unsaid words or actions within therapy (Worden, 2018). There is potential catharsis in simply verbalizing and exploring things they wished they had said or done. The client and therapist may also explore the client's thought distortions that emerge from such guilt or remorse and move potentially towards radical acceptance and forgiveness. Expressing what is unsaid or undone may help a client more effectively process their emotional responses to grief and prevent clinically significant complications.

GOAL

This process addresses the 1st, 2nd, and 3rd Task of Mourning. Its focus is for the client to communicate any thoughts or feelings they would like to have shared with the deceased. It provides an opportunity for them to identify any issues they may have had in their relationships that may have created barriers to effective grieving. This can further allow for future goal setting and treatment planning.

MATERIALS

Paper or canvas	Crayons
Paint	Magazine/book clippings
Markers/pens	Scissors
Color pencils	Glue
Pastels	Clay/Model Magic

INSTRUCTION

Ask the client to take some time to consider the things they would like to have said before their loss. What did they need to say? What words did they need to hear? Ask them not to censure these thoughts, but to consider all aspects of the unspoken conversation. When they are ready, ask them to create a piece around these unspoken words and their impact on them.

POSSIBLE PROCESSING QUESTIONS AND PROMPTS

After your client completes their piece, ask them to take time to reflect on what they have created. The following questions may be used to further explore the process.

1. Can you tell me about the piece you have created and how these unspoken conversations were expressed?

2. Can you share some of the things you wished you had been able to say before your loved one passed?

3. Can you share what you feel you needed to hear before their passing?

4. Why do you feel these words were important?

5. How did it feel to speak the unspoken now?

6. Of these unspoken words, which ones do you think have the greatest impact on you and your current grieving? Why?

7. How do you think your grief would be impacted now if you had been able to communicate the thoughts and feelings you have expressed here?

8. Did you notice any change in emotion between before and after the creation of your piece? What change did you notice?

9. How you do you think your grief will be impacted now that you have explored these unspoken words?

10. What steps do you think you can take to help you continue to process your grief?

FORGIVENESS

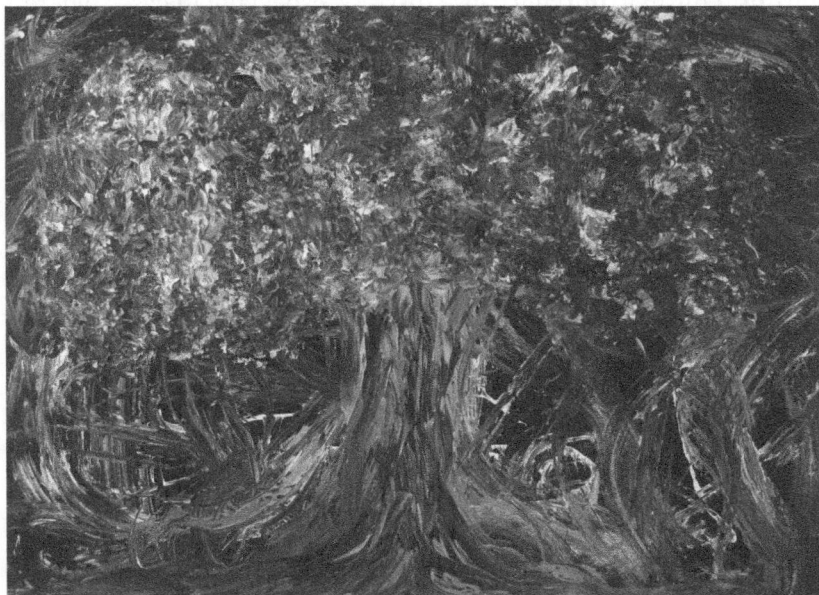

Figure 17: Forgiveness

PURPOSE

Shame, guilt, remorse, and anger are often elements of grief (Figley, 2013). Such feelings may evolve if unchecked, becoming self-attacks, eventually damaging self-efficacy and overall functioning. Losses that result in a great deal of shame may cause a severely damaged self-narrative, "and the only way back is through self-healing" (Figley, 2013, p.145). And perhaps the only way to achieve such self-healing is through forgiveness.

Forgiveness may also be necessary when the client feels anger or resentment if their relationship with the deceased was abusive or neglectful (Worden, 2018). This ties back to the *Things Left Unsaid* directive, in which sudden loss often leads to an inability to have needed conversations and closure.

Forgiveness can be complex and, at times, undesirable or avoided, but may be critical for effective grief processing. Forgiveness at its core "is the realization that one does not condone the transgressed acts or absolve responsibility, but it releases resentment" (Figley, 2013, p.145).

As the other party is now gone, forgiveness can only come from within. This may initially cause distress, especially in cases where a person realizes that the closure they long for will never occur (Figley, 2013). Forgiveness requires your client adjust their perspective from one of anger or shame to empathy and kindness. A person may best learn to accept the finality of the loss and reach a place of acceptance and self-love to continue their grieving journey.

GOAL

This process addresses the 2nd and 4th Task of Mourning. It asks the client to examine any unresolved issues or conflicts they had with the deceased. They may explore ambiguous loss, thought distortions, distress tolerance, and self-forgiveness. Additionally, this task may facilitate goal setting related to processing their conflicts with those they lost and find forgiveness within themselves.

MATERIALS

Paper or canvas	Crayons
Paint	Magazine/book clippings
Markers/pens	Scissors
Color pencils	Glue
Pastels	Clay/Model Magic

INSTRUCTION

Ask the client to consider any issues that they feel were left unaddressed and unresolved with the person who has died. Are they feeling shame or anger at themselves or the deceased? What would it look like to give/receive forgiveness? When they are ready, ask them to create a piece related to the idea of forgiveness and what it might feel like to forgive or be forgiven.

POSSIBLE PROCESSING QUESTIONS AND PROMPTS

After your client completes their piece, ask them to take time to reflect on what they have created. The following questions may be used to further explore the process.

1. Can you tell me about your piece? How does it represent forgiveness?

2. What feelings did you have while creating it? What feelings do you have looking at it now?

3. Can you tell me about the issues or topics you feel are unresolved?

4. How did it feel to consider these unresolved issues?

5. How do you feel these issues impacted your relationship with the deceased before their passing?

6. How do you think any unresolved issues have impacted your grieving process?

7. How did it feel to consider that only you can give and receive forgiveness now?

8. What would it mean to you to forgive?

9. How do you think forgiveness would change your grief?

10. How would it change your self-talk and self-esteem?

11. What steps do you think you could take to help you reach a place of forgiveness with either yourself, the deceased, or both?

CONTINUED CONNECTION

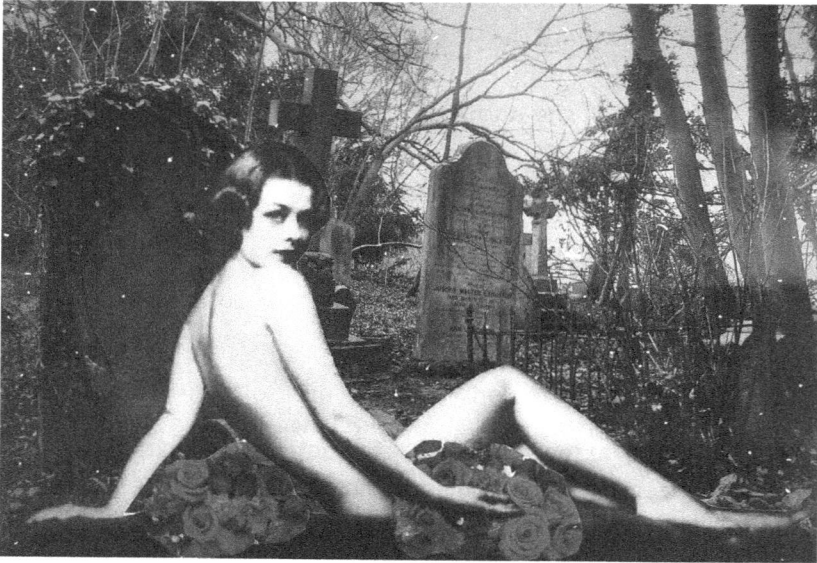

Figure 18: Continued Connection

PURPOSE

There was a time in the annals of grief counseling where complete emotional disconnection from the deceased was considered a marker of successful grieving (Klass, Silverman, & Nickman, 1999). Over the years, the realization dawned that this goal was not only impossible, but also a potentially unhealthy burden on the bereaved. The deceased continued to be connected to the bereaved through memories. For some, the memories and continued connections served to protect against complicated grief. These continued connections potentially lessened the impact of the death as it allowed the bereaved to continue to feel the presence of the deceased in their lives.

This continued connection with the dead is referred to as *continuing bonds* and may emerge in many ways (Worden, 2018). For instance, some clients continue to talk to their deceased loved ones.

Others may see signs of their loved one's continued presence through seemingly mystical experiences, such as finding feathers or pennies in odd places, often considered signs of the presence of the deceased (Jackson, 2020). Yet others may continue the bond with their loved one by setting up their pictures at holiday events. Such continuing bonds are specific for the client and their personal beliefs (Klass et al., 1999).

Still, for some, continuing bonds may become unhealthy (Klass et al., 1999), particularly if they are unable to work through the tasks of mourning because they become hyperfixated or obsessive on the connection. In such cases, the connection serves more as a barrier than a facilitator of effective grieving. Exploring these connections and their impact on the client may allow them to see the value or the detriment of their continuing bonds, allowing them to create goals to either strengthen or mitigate them, in turn assisting with therapeutic goal setting and emotional processing.

GOAL

The process may address the 1st and 3rd Task of Mourning. Its focus is to help the client explore their continuing bonds with the deceased and ways they may continue to feel connected to their loved one, or if unhealthy, mitigate the connection. This may lead them to eventually set goals towards meaning making and reintegration.

MATERIALS

Paper or canvas	Crayons
Paint	Magazine/book clippings
Markers/pens	Scissors
Color pencils	Glue
Pastels	Clay/Model Magic

INSTRUCTION

Ask the client to take a few moments to consider their connection to their loved one since they died. Do they still feel like their loved one is with them? What role do they see the deceased playing in their lives now? When they are ready, ask them to create a piece that represents the role of this connection in their lives.

POSSIBLE PROCESSING QUESTIONS AND PROMPTS

After your clients completes their piece, ask them to take time to reflect on what they have created. The following questions may be used to further explore the process.

1. Can you tell me about your piece and how it represents your current connection with the person you lost?

2. What are your beliefs about the ability to remain connected with someone who has died? How have these beliefs impacted your grief?

3. How important is it to continue to feel connected with your loved one? Why?

4. Have there been any experiences where you have felt the presence of your loved one? What happened? How did you feel after the experience?

5. Are there any actions you take to keep this connection? If so, what are the actions? How do you think these actions help you remain connected?

6. Do you feel like you want more of a connection to the deceased? Less? Why?

7. Are there any steps you could take that would help you reach your desired level of connection to the departed? What would these steps look like?

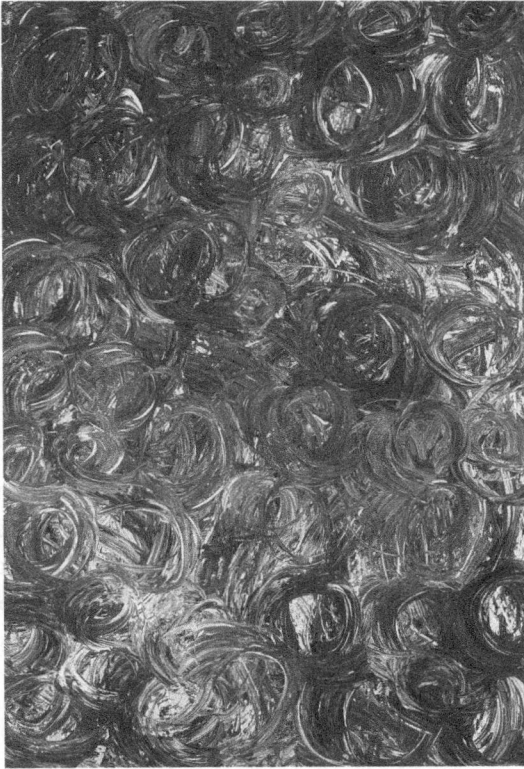

Figure 19: I Will Meet You There

PURPOSE

As outlined in the *Continuing Connections* directive, feeling a continuing bond with the deceased may aid in grieving and may protect against complicated grief. However, in some cases, a client may report feeling distress because they actually feel disconnected (Moss, 2005). In these cases, it may be beneficial to assist the client with developing a new connection with the deceased.

Moss (2005) is a spiritual practitioner who often counsels those that feel they need greater connection to their deceased loved one.

A technique he has found to be anecdotally helpful is to have the client imagine a place where they can "meet" with their loved one, a place that is either a real location where the client and the dead had previously interacted, or one imagined by the client. Moss then encourages his clients to meditate or imagine going to their place when they feel the need to talk with those they lost. Those who engage in this process have reporting experiencing less distress and greater feelings of connection.

This exercise is easily adapted to artistic creation and therapeutic practices. Adding an art-making element may help the client to concretize their imagined space thus strengthening their connection to the deceased. The place chosen or created for their "meeting" may also add insight into the relationship and allow for reminiscing or meaning making. These imagined meetings may also serve as a way for the client to increase feelings of closure by visualizing needed conversations or interactions.

GOAL

This process addresses the 1st, 2nd, and 3rd Task of Mourning. Asking your client to create a space to "meet" with their loved ones may provide an opportunity for increased feelings of connection and meaning making. This may lead them to eventually set goals towards reintegration, continuing into the 4th Task of Mourning.

MATERIALS

Paper or canvas	Crayons
Paint	Magazine/book clippings
Markers/pens	Scissors
Color pencils	Glue
Pastels	Clay/Model Magic

INSTRUCTION

Ask the client to consider their feeling of connection with the deceased. Do they feel they have a strong connection to their loved one since the passing? Weak? Ask them to consider places they spent time together in life. Then ask them to imagine a place where they could meet even now. What does this space look like? What does it feel like? What would they do in this safe meeting space? When they are ready, ask them to create this meeting space for them and their departed loved one.

POSSIBLE PROCESSING QUESTIONS AND PROMPTS

After your client completes their piece, ask them to take time to reflect on what they have created. The following questions may be used to further explore the process.

1. Can you tell me about your piece and the meeting space you have created?

2. Why did you choose this place? Did it have special meaning in life?

3. How did it feel to create a space for you and your loved one to "meet" even now?

4. If you were to meet them in this space, what would you say? What would you do?

5. How does this space make you feel?

6. Does this space change your feelings of connection to the departed? How?

7. When do you think you would visit this space, whether in thoughts or meditation?

8. How do you think visiting this space might impact your grief?

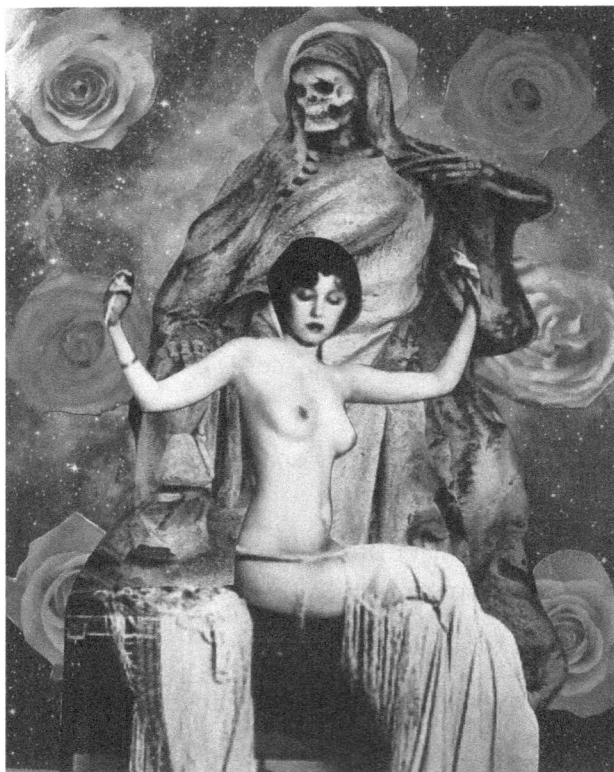

Figure 20: Dreaming of the Departed

PURPOSE

Dreaming of the deceased is common for the bereaved (Loconto, 1998). These dreams—their function and meaning—are often as unique as the client, and often contingent on a client's spiritual, religious, or cultural belief systems. For some, the dreams may be a sign of the continued connection to the deceased and beneficially serve their grieving (Wright et al., 2013). The dreams may allow the client an opportunity to interact with the deceased, further strengthening their bonds. For example, the dream may include replaying a cherished memory or a needed conversation that focuses on unfinished business (Wright et al., 2013).

There may also be instances where dreaming of the deceased causes distress (Hinton et al., 2013). For example, if the dreams include negative conversations or interactions, they may add to a client's feelings of anxiety or longing. Another example may be when the deceased was abusive towards the bereaved and this behavior was replayed in their dreams. If the dreams replay trauma, it may create sleep disturbances, becoming yet another barrier to effective grieving.

For still others, not dreaming of those they lost may also be a source of distress, feeling that the deceased is completely gone from their lives or is angry with them (Wright et al., 2013). Some, depending on their spiritual or religious beliefs, may even understand the lack of such dreams as a sign that their loved one has not yet "crossed over," causing further concern or distress.

Exploring dreams and their emotional impact on the client may aid in emotional processing and growing awareness of thought distortions. It may also aid in meaning making and goal setting.

GOAL

This process addresses the 1st, 2nd, and 3rd Task of Mourning. The client is prompted to consider any dreams they have had about their departed loved one and how these dreams—or lack thereof—may impact them and their grief. It may also provide an opportunity to challenge thought distortions and facilitate setting goals that focus on meaning making and reintegration.

MATERIALS

Paper or canvas	Crayons
Paint	Magazine/book clippings
Markers/pens	Scissors
Color pencils	Glue
Pastels	Clay/Model Magic

INSTRUCTION

Ask the client to consider any dreams they have had about their departed loved one since their passing. Are there any that stick out? If the dreams are recurring, have they noticed any themes? What were the feelings in the dream? When they woke up?

If the client has reported distress related to not dreaming about the deceased ask them to consider what this lack of dreaming means to them. What emotional responses is the lack of dreams creating within them?

When they are ready, ask them to create an image of a particular dream or their dreams as a whole.

POSSIBLE PROCESSING QUESTIONS AND PROMPTS

After your client completes their piece, ask them to reflect on what they created and consider the dream/dreams and the feelings associated with them. The following questions may be used to further explore the process.

1. Can you tell me about the piece you have created?

2. Can you tell me about your dream? What elements grabbed your attention or seemed important?

3. Was there any communication in the dream? Can you remember what was said?

4. How did you feel in the dream? Do you remember any emotional responses?

5. How did you feel when you when you woke up? What do you remember feeling physically? Emotionally?

6. How do you feel about dreaming about the deceased? Why?

7. How do you think your dream/dreams have impacted your grieving?

8. Do you think the dream is trying to communicate any unmet needs? If so, what do you think those needs are? How do you think you could meet those needs?

Figure 21: Reframing a
Nightmare 1

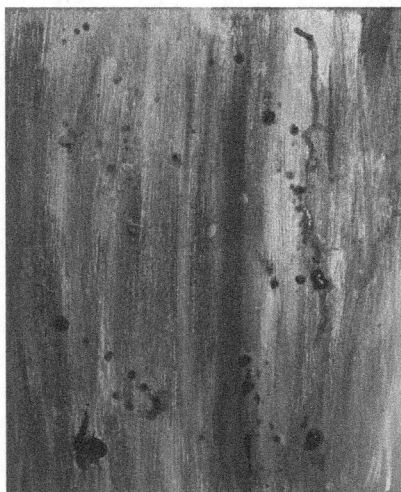

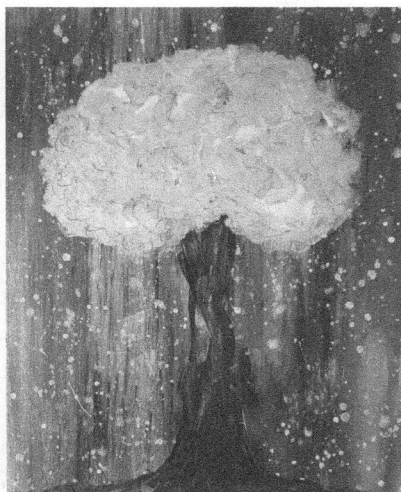

Figure 22: Reframing a
Nightmare 2

PURPOSE

As outlined in the *Dreaming of the Departed* directive, dreams are common in grieving. Such dreaming may take a darker turn, particularly when the loss is related to trauma; they may include reliving the event (Yucel et al., 2020). In cases where nightmares create significant distress; intervention may be necessary. A cycle may be created where the person has difficulty staying asleep due to the nightmares, in turn impairing their ability to function during the day from lack of sleep, creating yet further difficulty falling asleep out of a fear of the nightmare's return. If left unaddressed, these sleep disturbances may create a risk for complicated grief (Worden, 2018).

A variety for treatment options have been explored in treating nightmares associated with trauma; the most empirically supported seems to be image reversal therapy (IRT: Krakow & Zadra, 2006). IRT is a cognitive behavioral visualization technique where the client is asked to review their nightmares and then create a new ending for the dream (Yucel et al., 2020). It is understood that this technique may help by removing the power from the dream and returning it to the dreamer.

As with other discussed visualization techniques, IRT seems to be easily adapted to an art-based technique. By allowing the client to depict the nightmare and its new ending in a visual form, it helps it become more tangible and controllable. This may alleviate sleep disturbances and aid emotional processing to facilitate effective grieving. It may also increase feelings of self-efficacy and hope.

GOAL

This process addresses the 1st, 2nd, and 3rd Task of Mourning. Its focus is to help clients regain a sense of control over their sleep by examining and reframing any distressing nightmares. It is also anticipated that such an examination will help reduce any fear, anxiety, or distress a client may be feeling around nightmares, eventually contributing to better-quality sleep. It may also facilitate new goals to improve sleep and thus overall functioning.

MATERIALS

Paper or canvas	Crayons
Paint	Magazine/book clippings
Markers/pens	Scissors
Color pencils	Glue
Pastels	Clay/Model Magic

INSTRUCTION

This process is intended to be completed over two sessions to allow for full exploration. In the second part, the client will be covering/changing the image so consider this when selecting the materials.

Once completed refer to the Part 1 processing questions and prompts before moving to Part 2.

Part 1

Ask the client to take a few moments to consider recent or recurring nightmares that are causing them distress and impacting their sleep. What is happening in the nightmare? Are there certain people present? How does the nightmare impact their sleep and emotions? When they are ready, ask them to create a visual representation of this nightmare.

Part 2

Ask the client to spend a few moments viewing their creation from Part 1 and to consider how they would change it. What would make the nightmare less scary? How could they change the nightmare to feel a sense of power over it? When they are ready, ask them to cover the image of the nightmare with a new image that they find beautiful, hopeful, or inspiring. This image may relate to the discussion around the original image and what it is trying to communicate.

POSSIBLE PROCESSING QUESTIONS AND PROMPTS
Part 1

1. Can you tell me about your creation and your nightmare? How did it feel to think about this nightmare? To visually create it?

2. If this dream could talk, what do you think it would say?

3. How do you think the nightmare relates to your grief and loss?

4. As you were considering the nightmare, were there any elements of it that stood out to you? Why or why not?

5. When you had this nightmare, how did you feel in the dream? When you woke up?

6. Do you think this nightmare has impacted your sleep? If so, how?

7. How do you feel about the nightmare now that you have

drawn/painted it? Have those feelings changed from before the drawing/painting?

8. Are there any steps you take to reduce the emotional impact of the nightmare?

Part 2

1. Can you tell me about the piece you have created and how it shows your new dream? Are there any elements that stick out to you? Why?

2. What do you think this new dream image is saying?

3. How do you feel when you look at your new dream? How is this different from the previous nightmare?

4. How do you feel about the nightmare now that you have changed it?

5. Have your feelings of fear or anxiety changed? If so, how do you think these changes will impact your sleep?

6. Is there anything from this experience of changing a nightmare that might help you in the future? If so, how?

7. How do you think altering this nightmare may impact your grief?

THEN AND NOW

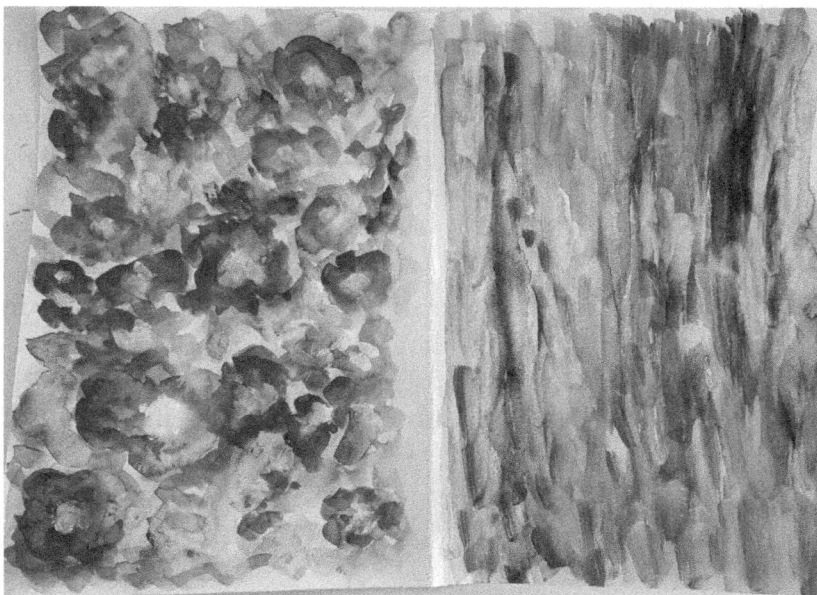

Figure 23: Then and Now

PURPOSE

Loss and trauma can create an emotional line in a person's life demarcating the perceived time before the loss and after (Palgi et al., 2018). The time before is often perceived in an idealistic, positive way and the time after as negative. Such perception can create increased despair in the client as they long for the perfection of the time before their loss and struggle to find the positive after.

Viewing the past and present in such distorted and inaccurate extremes may have a negative impact on grieving and overall functioning (Palgi et al., 2018). For example, a client who experienced a hysterectomy may describe her life before the surgery as hopeful and happy without acknowledging the pain and trauma her failing uterus had caused her. Since she is not acknowledging the negative of the before, she may experience more sadness and longing after.

Clients who view the loss in such extremes may experience increased distress, longing, and hopelessness. Those that maintain distorted perceptions of their time before the loss as so perfect, often believe they may never hope to have that level of perfection again. This can erect a barrier to reintegration, making it difficult to move forward in life.

To assist the client with their continued grief processing it may be necessary to explore their perceptions of the time before their loss compared to their present life and functioning. This may allow for reality orientation and offer a means to challenge such emerging thought distortions.

GOAL

This process may address the 3rd Task of Mourning. Its focus is to help a client identify possible thought distortions and reality testing related to their perceptions of life before and after their loss. It further promotes goal formation around increasing self-efficacy and mastery.

MATERIALS

Paper or canvas	Crayons
Paint	Magazine/book clippings
Markers/pens	Scissors
Color pencils	Glue
Pastels	Clay/Model Magic

INSTRUCTION

Ask the client to take a moment to reflect on their lives before their loss. What did this life look like? Feel like? Then ask then to consider their life now. How does this new life look and feel? How are these two lives similar? Different? When they are ready, provide the client with a piece of paper that you have folded in half and ask them to create an image of their "before" life on the left side and the "after" life on the right side.

POSSIBLE PROCESSING QUESTIONS AND PROMPTS

After your client completes their piece, ask them to reflect on what they created and consider the aspects and feelings of their two "lives." The following questions may be used to further explore the process.

1. Can you describe your "before" image? Your "after"?

2. What stands out most in the two images? Why?

3. How do you feel your life has changed from your loss?

4. If you could assign one word to each picture, what would that word be? What does that word mean to you?

5. Do you think these images are accurate representations of your before and after life? Why or why not?

6. How do you feel you have changed as a person from before the loss to now? How do you feel about these changes? Are these changes represented in your creation? How?

7. Are there any areas in the images you would like to change? Why?

8. Are there any aspects of your life now that you would like to change? What are they? What steps could you take to create this change?

THE MARK THEY MADE

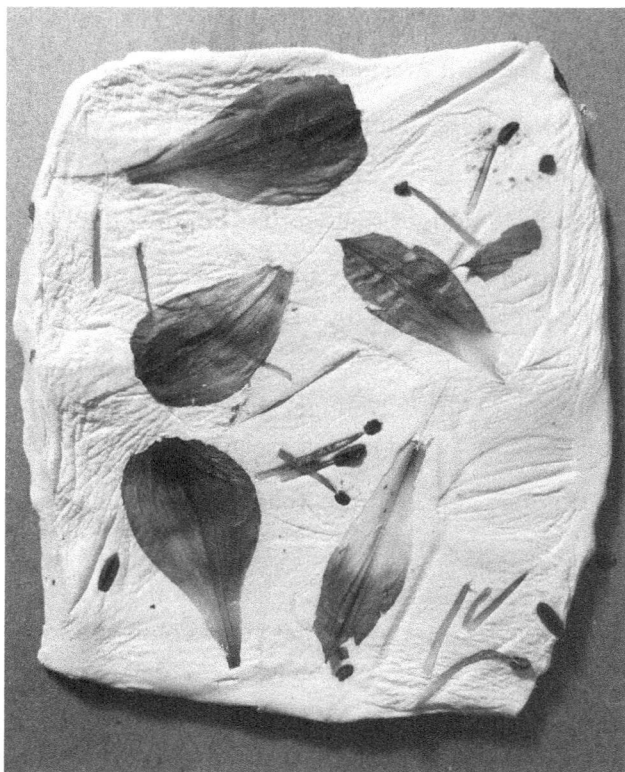

Figure 24: The Mark They Made

PURPOSE

As indicated in the *Memories* directive, being able to reminisce and share stories of the deceased benefits a person's grieving process (Worden, 2018). As a person works through their grief, they may reach a point where it would be helpful for the person to consider not only the memories of the deceased, but also explore the specific impact the deceased had upon their lives.

The 4th Task of Mourning asks the client not only to remember the departed, but also to become more action-focused (Worden,

2018). The client is asked to decide how they can keep the memory and impact of the deceased present in their lives while moving forward, creating a more future-focused impact. It also returns feelings of power and control to those who are experiencing the loss by encouraging them to make active decisions on how they will allow the loss to impact their future.

This may be more complex in cases of conflicted relationships (Rando, 1984). In such cases, the impact the deceased had on the client may not always have been positive. The person may begin to experience feelings of helplessness, believing they carry the burden of the negative effects the deceased left behind (Worden, 2018), becoming a potential risk for complicated grief.

While it is true that a person had no control over the role the deceased played in their life, they have a choice about how it impacts their future. By facilitating the client's reflections, they may develop awareness of the power they actually have over the deceased's impact on their own lives, facilitating feelings of mastery and empowerment (Worden, 2018), eventually allowing for further emotional processing and future goal setting.

GOAL

This process may address the 4th Task of Mourning. Its focus is to help a client reflect on how the departed impacted their lives, either positively or negatively, promoting decision making on what they want to hold on to and what they would like to move beyond. It further provides opportunities to formulate goals on identifying desired changes on just what the lasting impact of the deceased will be.

MATERIALS

Air dry clay

Found objects

Rolling pin

Objects from nature
(flowers, sticks, rocks)

INSTRUCTION

*Before this session, ask the client to collect objects that represent the impact their loved one had on their lives. For example, if the person felt the departed was reliable, maybe they could gather stones, or if conflictual, maybe dirt or ashes.

Ask the client to reflect on the relationship they had with the departed. How do they feel about the relationship? How did this relationship impact their lives and change them, their thoughts, and their beliefs? When they are ready, ask the client to shape the clay into a flat surface in whatever shape feels right to them. When the clay is flat, ask them to place the objects they have collected onto the clay and press them in. They can use the rolling pin to help press and smooth the objects. It is up to them whether they leave the objects embedded in the clay or if they remove them and only leave the imprint of the object.

POSSIBLE PROCESSING QUESTIONS AND PROMPTS

After your client has completed their piece, ask them to consider how the clay changed from a blank, smooth surface to what it became after adding the objects. Ask them to reflect on how this clay is similar to themselves and the departed. The following questions may be used to further explore the process.

1. Can you tell me about the piece you created? The objects you selected?

2. How did you decide which pieces to leave in the clay and which ones to remove?

3. Can you share how you feel the departed impacted your life as a whole?

4. What are some specific ways you are still impacted?

5. Do you think the piece you created shows this impact? How or how not?

6. How did it feel to create this piece? To see that some things

once they were imprinted were easy/difficult to remove? How do you think this relates to you?

7. What things did the departed leave with you that you would like to keep?

8. What elements do you think you need to leave behind? If any, how do you think you could accomplish this?

9. As you go into your future, what steps can you take to incorporate into your life the elements you have chosen to keep? How do you think this will impact your grieving?

THE INNER ROOM DIORAMA

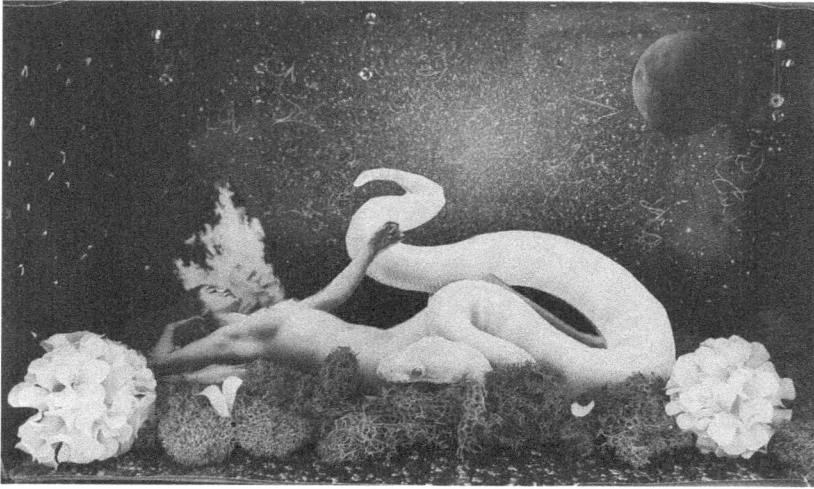

Figure 25: The Inner Room Diorama (created inside a shoe box)

PURPOSE

When a person experiences a loss, they often express a physical or emotional void where what was lost used to be (Worden, 2018). In some cases, the void can be quite literal, such as a newly empty seat at the dinner table or an empty internal space where a cancerous organ used to be. In other cases, the void may be more intangible. Bereaved clients often indicate feeling empty or that their lives feel empty.

There are many ways for a client to visualize and describe this void. Conceptualizing the void as a physical room may help a person inventory what has been lost and how it has impacted their life. This review may help the client acknowledge what was lost, how their lives have changed, and how they can repurpose or change this vacant space within themselves as the go into the future. This directive aims to assist the client in reviewing and acknowledging what was lost while becoming empowered to create new and positive changes within themselves and their lives.

A word of caution when working with the concept of the physical aspect of a loss: there is a risk of increasing distress in a client if the focus is placed on filling the void instead of restructuring it. In such cases, depending on how it is presented, it may cause a person to feel as if they are not whole and may never be whole again because of their loss. Focusing on filling the void instead of restructuring or adapting to it may increase such feelings, thus increasing hopelessness and helplessness. The goal is to encourage feelings of wholeness and self-efficacy despite the loss, not replacing it.

GOAL

This process may address the 3rd and 4th Task of Mourning. It focuses on exploring the space that was left in their lives after they experienced their loss. Doing so may increase feelings of mastery and control, further providing an opportunity to create new goals that focus on life restructuring and future planning.

MATERIALS

Small box (e.g., shoe box)	Glue
Paint	Scissors
Markers	Found objects
Magazine/book clippings	

INSTRUCTION

Ask the client to take a moment to reflect on the space the lost person or item once held in their lives and within themselves. Ask them to picture this as a room. What did this room look like? What did the room feel like? Keeping this imagery of the room in mind, ask the client to picture that room now. What does it look like? How has the feeling of the room changed? When they are ready, ask the client to create a diorama showing what their inner room looks like now using the materials provided.

*This directive could be completed in three parts with a diorama created for the room before the loss, after the loss, and in the future.

POSSIBLE PROCESSING QUESTIONS AND PROMPTS

After the client completes their rooms, ask them to reflect on them. The following questions may be used to further explore the process.

1. Can you tell me what your inner room looked like before your loss? How did this room make you feel?

2. Can you tell me about the piece you have created? How does this new room make you feel?

3. How is this room different from the room before your loss?

4. How do you feel viewing this "now" room?

5. Have your feelings about this room changed from when you first pictured it in your mind to now when you are viewing it externally? How so?

6. If you could describe this room in one word, what would it be? What does this word mean to you?

7. What do you view as positive aspects of the room you have created? Negative?

8. Are there any changes you would like to make to this room? If so, what actions do you think you need to take to create this change?

9. How would you like this room to look in the future? What steps could you take to create this future room?

MOURNING THE FUTURE

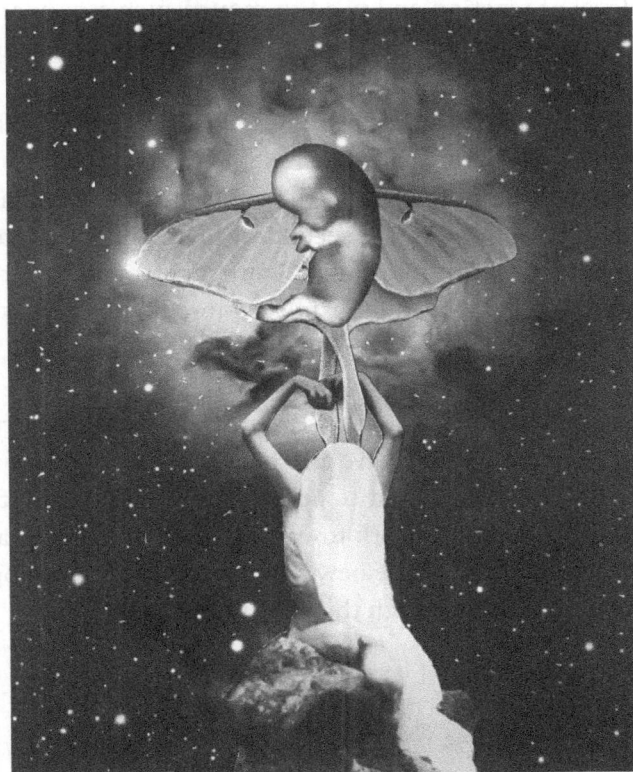

Figure 26: Mourning the Future

PURPOSE

Secondary losses refer to losses that occur as a result of the original one, often occurring in the future (Rando, 1984). These losses are not always immediately apparent and tend to appear over time as the full scope of the loss is considered and processed. For example, when a loved one dies, a person will not only grieve the death, but also future experiences that will never be shared, such as weddings, graduations, or the birth of children.

Secondary losses not only occur when someone has died but

emerge in other types of losses as well (Doka, 2002). For example, if a man has gone through a divorce, he may grieve the retirement and travel plans he shared with his ex-wife. If there were children involved, he may grieve the reduced time he is allowed to spend with his children and the memories he is unable to make with them.

The level of reaction and need to mourn such secondary losses will be dependent on the level of meaning or type of attachment that existed for the one experiencing the loss (Worden, 2018). If a woman never desired children, she may not grieve a hysterectomy. In some cases, she may actually feel joy and relief. If the divorced woman felt her husband was holding her back in life, she may celebrate her new-found freedom. For others, the secondary losses may be as painful as the original loss—if not more so. As with all elements of grief, it is unique to the individual and must be explored without bias.

GOAL

This process may address all four Tasks of Mourning. It focuses on exploring what future may have also been lost as a result of the primary loss. It allows the client to acknowledge and mourn this lost future, allowing them to work towards successful reintegration. It may further help them create new goals around different hopes and actions they can take to reach this new future.

MATERIALS

Paper or canvas	Crayons
Paint	Magazine/book clippings
Markers/pens	Scissors
Color pencils	Glue
Pastels	Clay/Model Magic

INSTRUCTION

Ask the client to consider what hopes or plans were also lost when they experienced the loss causing their current grief. What did that future look like? What did they dream of accomplishing that they now feel they cannot? When they are ready, ask them to create a piece about this lost future.

POSSIBLE PROCESSING QUESTIONS AND PROMPTS

After your client completes their piece, ask them to reflect on it. The following questions may be used to further explore the process.

1. Can you tell me about your piece and the lost future you have chosen to depict?

2. Had you previously considered this aspect of loss in your grieving? How do you feel it has impacted your grief?

3. How did it feel to create a piece about this part of your grief? Did you notice any changes in your mood or body?

4. If you could assign one word to this element of your grief what would that word be? What does that word mean to you?

5. How much do you think these unmet future hopes are impacting your current grieving?

6. Have you considered any new hopes or dreams? If you have, what does this new future look like?

7. If you haven't considered a new future before now, what would you like to see in your life as you move forward?

8. What steps could you take to help you reach your new goals?

SAYING GOODBYE

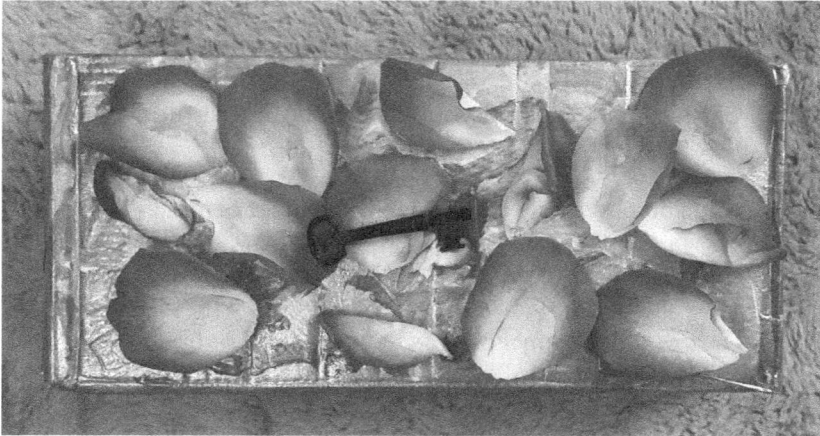

Figure 27: Saying Goodbye

PURPOSE

Funerals are necessary for the grieving process, and potentially can prevent complicated grief (Rando, 1984; Worden, 2018), as they "become the vehicle by which grief is acknowledged and sanctioned and in which support is extended" (Doka, 2002, p.9). Still, some may be unable to attend for a variety of reasons, such as being unable to afford traveling such a long distance, or illness may prevent them from being able to attend, common during the COVID-19 pandemic (Kokou-Kpolou, Fernández-Alcántara, & Cénat, 2020). Other times, in cases of disenfranchised grief, the one grieving may not be welcome at the funeral (Doka, 2002); particularly in situations of infidelity, divorce, or family conflicts; simply put, they may have been excluded from being allowed to participate in this necessary ritual, creating even more difficulties.

One new trend is that rather than a traditional funeral, for whatever reason, the deceased is remembered in a celebration of life service (Worden, 2018). Such a ceremony emphasizes the joy of a person's life and encourages mourners to feel positively towards the deceased, eschewing the sadness typical of such traditional ceremonies. In most of these ceremonies, the deceased's body is not present or is present in the form of cremated remains.

While these ceremonies can be well intentioned, they may serve to disenfranchise normal grief reactions and create obstacles to undergoing the first two Tasks of Mourning. Focusing on the positive emotions may cause those who are feeling deep sadness and despair to believe that their reactions to the death are inappropriate or unseen (Worden, 2018). In addition, seeing the body of the deceased may help the bereaved accept the loss more quickly; when the body is not available for viewing, there is a risk of the bereaved convincing themselves that their loved one is not truly gone. When a funeral is not conducted, it may be necessary to engage in an alternative, symbolic ceremony. This may aid the client's acceptance of the loss and facilitate the opportunity for communal support.

GOAL

This process may address the 1st and 2nd Task of Mourning. Its focus is to assist a client with accepting the death, expressing emotions, and meaning making. It can further allow for death acceptance and reintegration.

MATERIALS

Small box or large white envelope	Found objects (flowers, trinkets, rocks, etc.)
Paint	Pictures
Markers	Glue
Color pencils/pens	

INSTRUCTION

Ask the client to think of the deceased and what they would have liked to say at a funeral to memorialize them. What memories come up for them? What did they add to their life? Was there a certain story they would have liked to share? When they are ready, ask them to decorate either a small box or large envelope as a memorial to the departed. When they have finished decorating, ask them to write a letter/eulogy.

After processing, ask the client to place the letter inside the box/envelope and dispose of it in a way they choose (e.g., burial, burning, throwing it away, keeping it on a shelf). Adjustments to this directive should be made to fit the specific cultural and spiritual beliefs of the client.

POSSIBLE PROCESSING QUESTIONS AND PROMPTS

After your client completes their piece, ask them to take time to consider the memorial vessel they have created and the letter they have written. If they are comfortable, ask them to read the letter out loud. The following questions may be used to further explore the process.

1. How did it feel to be unable to attend/hold a funeral for your loved one?

2. Do you think it impacted your grieving? If so, how?

3. How important was it for you to have your own funeral? Why?

4. How did this experience as a whole feel? Creating the memorial box/envelope? Writing the letter?

5. If you could describe this experience with one word, what would that word be? What does that word mean to you?

6. Did this experience change any of the feelings you identified you experienced from not having a funeral? How?

7. Do you think this experience will change your grieving process going forward? How?

ANNIVERSARY

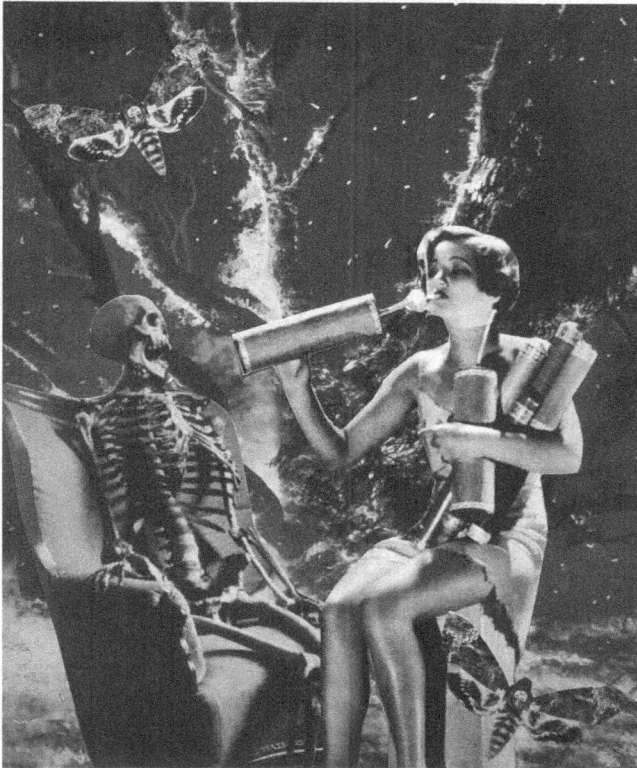

Figure 28: Anniversary

PURPOSE

As someone works through their loss, there may be times of the year that were significant for the deceased, and/or relationship which may create more acute grief than other days (Chow, 2009). These may include birthdays, wedding anniversaries and other holidays that were meaningful. During these times, a client may report greater longing or sadness, perhaps impacting their daily functioning yet again.

The anniversary of the death may be particularly difficult and triggering, particularly in cases of complicated or unprocessed grief (Worden, 2018). If the death was traumatic, there may be increased distress through intrusive thoughts and nightmares.

Some report heightened substance usage/abuse and suicidal feelings as they approach the death anniversary, as seen in a study conducted by Hiyoshi et al. (2022) for both male and female participants in the month preceding, month of, and month after the anniversary. However, these are most significant for the first anniversary, decreasing over subsequent years.

Taking this into consideration, it may be critical to begin planning for coping strategies well in advance of the death anniversary. Early intervention may allow the therapist to help the client identify systems that can provide extra support if needed. They may also be able to identify techniques that can be used if emotions become overwhelming. This may help minimize the risks and facilitate continued grief processing.

GOAL

This process may address the 2nd and 4th Task of Mourning. By asking the client to explore their feelings related to the upcoming death anniversary, it promotes strategies to help gain and sustain support that may help mitigate the increased emotional response to the anniversary.

MATERIALS

Paper or canvas	Crayons
Paint	Magazine/book clippings
Markers/pens	Scissors
Color pencils	Glue
Pastels	Clay/Model Magic

INSTRUCTION

Ask the client to reflect on the upcoming death anniversary. How are they feeling as the day approaches? What emotions are they seeing an increase in? When they are ready, ask them to create a piece representing their feelings about this approaching day and its impact on them and their grief.

POSSIBLE PROCESSING QUESTIONS AND PROMPTS

After your client completes their piece, ask them to take some time to reflect on it. The following questions may be used to further explore the process.

1. Can you tell me about your artwork and how it represents your feelings about the upcoming anniversary?

2. How are you feeling emotionally as you consider the anniversary? Physically?

3. Are there any emotions/behaviors that you are seeing an increase in? What are they? How are they impacting your grief?

4. If this piece could talk, what do you think it would say?

5. Are there any actions you are taking to help you prepare for this day? If so, what are they?

6. Are there any things that you think would make this day easier for you to handle emotionally? Any things you feel you need to avoid on that day?

7. What skills do you think would be helpful if you begin to feel overwhelmed on the anniversary?

8. Do you have a support system in place to help you during this day? How do you think this support may be helpful? Are those who give you support aware of your possible need for extra support on this day?

9. How will you know when you need to reach out for support? How comfortable do you feel asking for support?

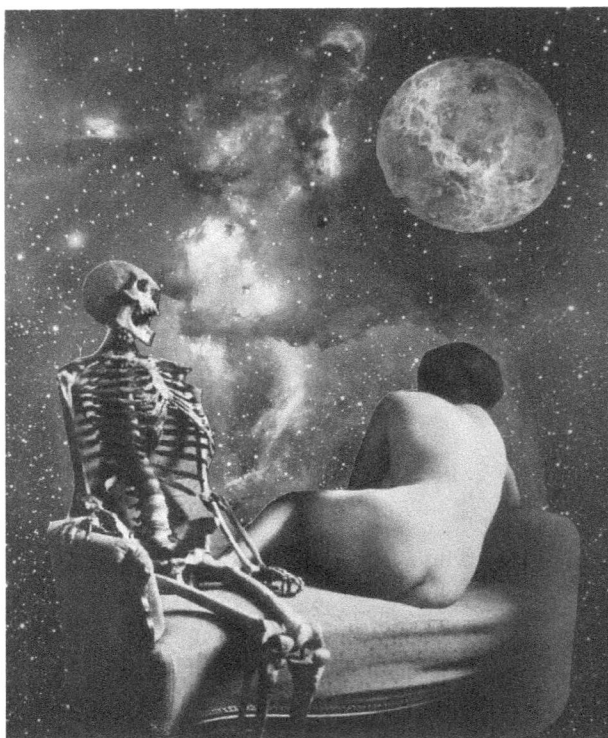

Figure 29: Labels

PURPOSE

A person who has experienced a loss will often identify with new self-labels. These labels may come from within or be assigned to them by society, such as, widow, survivor, or victim (Doka, 2002). While these may create a sense of connection with others who have experienced a similar loss, there is also the potential for the label to become limiting by overidentifying with an attached stigma (Kenney, 2002). There is a risk that a person may begin to feel as though they have lost their previous identity and have now become this given or adopted label (Farrington, 2014).

Still, others may inspire or help an individual make meaning from their loss (Farrington, 2014). The label of survivor may promote hope or propel one towards activism and community engagement. For example, a person who is labeled a "cancer survivor" may become active in fundraisers and community groups that focus on this medical condition.

However, there remains the risk that a person may experience a decrease of self-efficacy as they adopt real or imagined limitations connected to their new label (Worden, 2018). Some may feel they are treated differently after their loss, which may, in time, become self-fulfilling as they adjust to a new mentality congruent with how others perceive or treat them. For example, a widow begins to take on more helpless and dependent responses as those around her treat her as emotionally fragile.

Creating a balance between their new labels and their sense of agency is critical, as succumbing to dependent and one-dimensional labels increases the possibility of complicated grief (Worden, 2018). By exploring the client's views on any new labels they have adopted or have been given by those around them, they may gain new insight into how the label may be impacting their grief process.

GOAL
This process addresses the 2nd Task of Mourning. Its focus is to help a client explore their new label(s) and how it may be impacting them. This may further aid in balancing self-identity and self-integration.

MATERIALS

Paper or canvas	Crayons
Paint	Magazine/book clippings
Markers/pens	Scissors
Color pencils	Glue
Pastels	Clay/Model Magic

INSTRUCTION

Ask the client to take a few moments and consider any new labels they have been given or adopted since their loss. What does the label mean to them? How much to they relate to the label? When they are ready, ask them to create a piece that represents their label and their feelings towards it.

POSSIBLE PROCESSING QUESTIONS AND PROMPTS

After your client completes their piece, ask them to reflect on their creation and consider their ideas about how they are portrayed. The following questions may be used to further explore the process.

1. Can you tell me about your creation and the label you focused on?

2. What are your thoughts about this label? What does it mean to be a [insert label]?

3. How are these thoughts represented in your art?

4. What are your own beliefs about being a [insert label]?

5. If you had to assign one word to your feelings about this label, what would that word be?

6. How do you feel this label is impacting you? Your grief?

7. Are there any aspects the label that you feel are a barrier to your grieving? Are there are aspects of the label that you find helpful?

8. How much do you feel you identify with the label?

9. Do you think your level of self-identification with the label is beneficial? Harmful?

10. Are there any changes you would like to see with how you relate to the label? What would those changes look like? How do you think they would impact your grief? Your life in general?

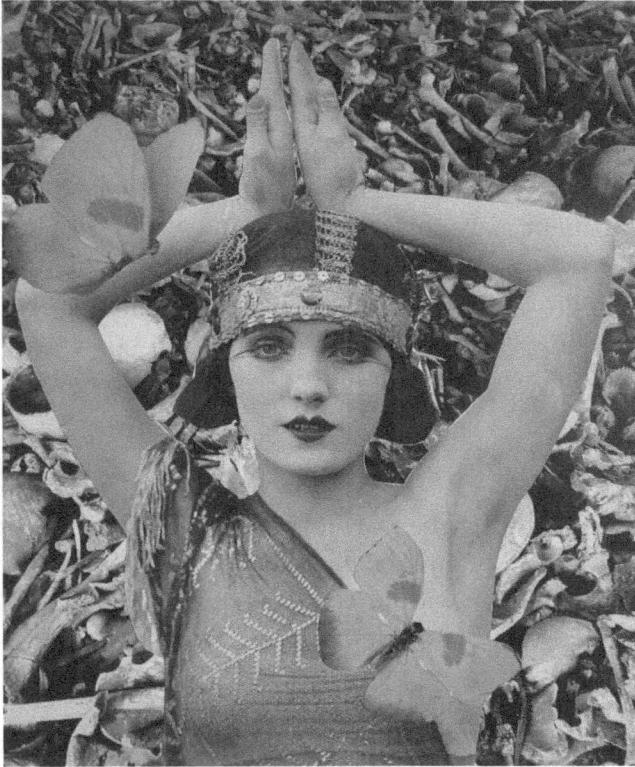

Figure 30: Inside Outside

PURPOSE

For many people, their setting influences how they perceive themselves and may inform how they act or even "who they are." A person at home may be quite different from the person they are at work. While this is normal in most cases, congruent with the tenets of *interactionism* (Blumer, 1969; James, 1890/1918; Mead, 1964), in grief work this may be a symptom of "masked grief reactions" or simply *masking* (Worden, 2018). This can result in complications, sometimes manifesting into complicated grief. "If a person does not express

145

feelings in an overt manner, this unmanifested grief will be expressed completely in some other way" (Worden, 2018, p.147).

When grief is not identified and processed, it may increase depression, somatic symptoms, such as pain, or other maladaptive behaviors and reactions, such as substance abuse (Worden, 2018) and suicidality. The person is unable or unwilling to relate these symptoms or behaviors to their latent grief. In such extreme cases, their grief becomes blocked, increasing the likelihood of complicated grief.

It is critical to help a client realign and acknowledge the internal grief process that may be impacting them. "Once the therapist helps the patient make this connection and works with him or her to identify and resolve the underlying separation conflicts, there is a decided improvement in the physical and/or mental symptoms" (Worden, 2018, p.149). By helping someone's internal and external world realign, they may have more effective emotional processing and behaviors.

GOAL

This process addresses the 2nd and 3rd Task of Mourning. Its focus is to help the client examine the self they show the world versus the one they keep hidden within. This may help a client identify their needs and how they may better align their inner and outer selves.

MATERIALS

Paper or canvas	Crayons
Paint	Magazine/book clippings
Markers/pens	Scissors
Color pencils	Glue
Pastels	Clay/Model Magic

INSTRUCTION

Ask the client to take a few moments to think about the person they show the world. Who are they when they are with friends or family?

Who are they when they feel supported versus unsupported? Now ask them to consider how they feel internally? Who is the person that they hide from others? What emotions have they hidden? When they are ready, ask them to create a piece that shows both their inner and outer world in one image.

POSSIBLE PROCESSING QUESTIONS AND PROMPTS

After your client completes their piece, ask them to take time to reflect on what they have created. The following questions may be used to further explore the process.

1. Can you tell me about your art as a whole?

2. Can you tell me about the inner world you depicted? The outer world?

3. How do these two worlds interact? How is this shown in your art?

4. If you could assign one word to the person you show the world, what would it be? To the inner person? What does each of these words mean to you?

5. How are your inner and outer people different? How are they similar?

6. What aspects from your inner world are not being expressed? Why?

7. Did you notice any changes between your inner and outer worlds after your loss?

8. How do you think that has impacted your grief?

9. What do you think these unexpressed aspects of you need? How would you be more comfortable expressing them? What steps could you take to meet these needs?

10. Are there any changes you would like to make to align your inner and outer worlds? How do you think you could accomplish these changes?

TRUE SELF, SOUL PORTRAIT

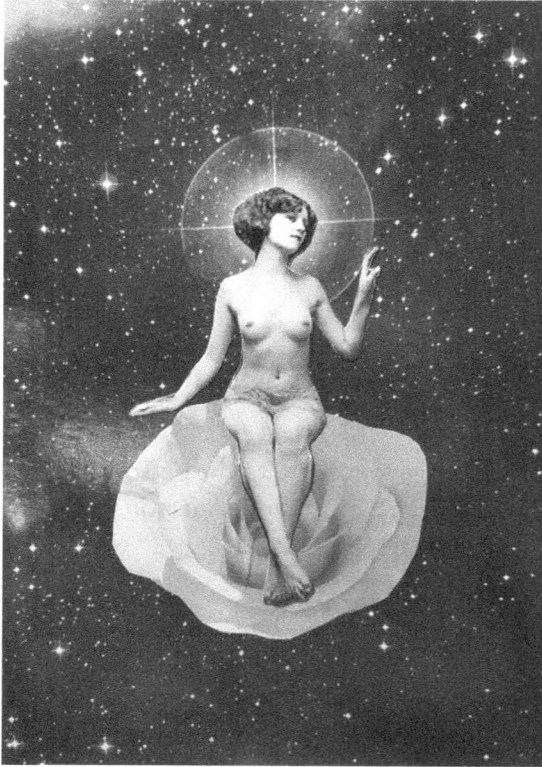

Figure 31: True Self, Soul Portrait

PURPOSE

As indicated in the *Labels* directive, it is not uncommon after losing someone to either adopt or be given a new identity that underscores the loss, such as, widow, survivor, or victim (Rando, 1984). While these new labels may be helpful, they could also pose a risk of becoming a dominant identifier, cancelling out other aspects of the self (Charland, 2004). For example, a woman whose husband died is known as "widow," whereas before his death she considered herself as a mother, an artist, and an adventurer. In essence, her new label cancelled out the other ways she saw herself.

If such a thing happens, it may be a sign that they have lost touch with, or turned away from, the other aspects of themselves (Worden, 2018). Perhaps the newly identified "widow" stopped creating the art that she loved or has stopped hiking in favor of only those events that focus on her loss, or she finds herself becoming more dependent on others. While there is nothing inherently wrong with this, it may reflect an imbalance and over-identification.

Helping a client reconnect with the other important parts of themselves may be crucial to successful reintegration and increase feelings of self-efficacy and power. Further, a more holistic sense of self may aid in effective grieving by creating a sense of balance, which could serve as a protective factor against complicated grief (Worden, 2018).

GOAL

This process addresses the 3rd and 4th Task of Mourning. Its focus is to help a client view who they are in addition to the loss they have experienced. It provides an opportunity to examine attributes about themselves that make them unique and increase self-confidence, self-efficacy, and mastery. This examination can allow for goal formation around self-care and related tasks.

MATERIALS

Paper or canvas	Crayons
Paint	Magazine/book clippings
Markers/pens	Scissors
Color pencils	Glue
Pastels	Clay/Model Magic

INSTRUCTION

Ask the client to take a few moments and consider who they are at their core beyond their current loss and grief. Ask them to think about the characteristics that they identify as *self*. How would they describe themselves to others? It may help for them to make a list of characteristics before completing the art creation. After they have considered or listed these characteristics, ask the client to create an image to represent this truest self, their soul.

POSSIBLE PROCESSING QUESTIONS AND PROMPTS

After your client completes their piece, ask them to take time to reflect on what they created considering their identified characteristics and how they are portrayed. The following questions may be used to further explore the process.

1. Can you tell me about your art and how it reflects you?

2. Could you tell me some characteristics of your true self?

3. How did you represent these characteristics in your piece?

4. How do you feel when you look at this image? What sticks out the most?

5. How much of this true self do you currently show to the world? Why?

6. What does it mean to be true to yourself?

7. Do you feel your personal identity between your grief and non-grief self is balanced? How do you feel it is balanced? How do you feel it is unbalanced?

8. What characteristics do you feel you have gained through your grief? Which have you lost?

9. Are there any characteristics that you would like to see more of? Less of? How could you accomplish this?

10. What steps do you think you could take to acknowledge all aspects of your self? How do you think this would impact your life and your grief?

MY MORTALITY

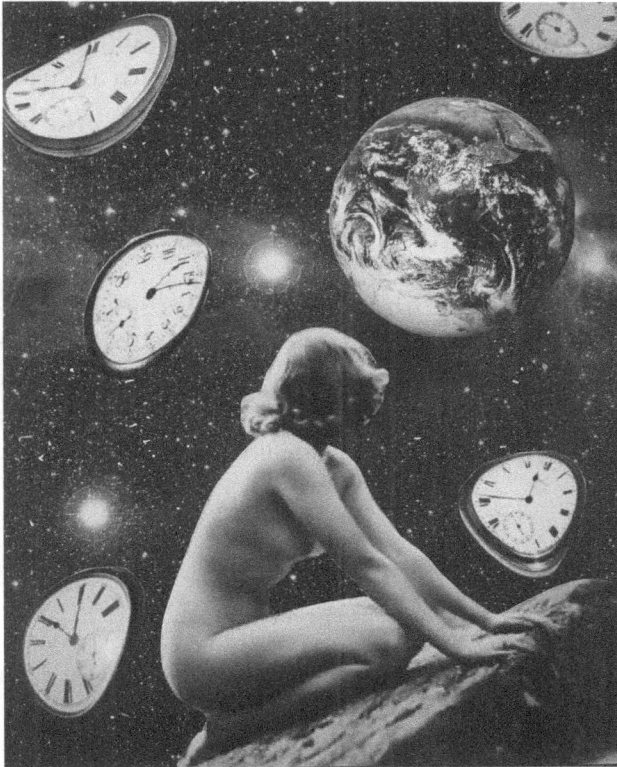

Figure 32: My Mortality

PURPOSE

Death brings existential concerns for the bereaved (Yalom, 1980), as a person not only processes the death, but the idea of their own mortality as well. "Mortality has haunted us from the beginning of history" (Yalom, 2009, p.1). When someone is confronted with death, either of someone close to them or when diagnosed with their own life-threatening illness, they often find themselves contemplating their own impermanence.

For some, the idea of their finite existence is overwhelming, creating "death anxiety," wherein they begin to act in maladaptive ways that seem to deny their own mortality. For example, after experiencing the death of a friend, a young man begins to participate in risk-taking behaviors in an attempt to fight against death and his own mortality.

Considering one's own mortality is expected and is necessary for effective grieving and preventing potential death anxiety (Yalom, 2009). Some who fear their own death may feel like their life is meaningless and hopeless; others may come to fear the loss of people who they are close to and begin to isolate to ward off future pain. Self-isolation could reduce or eliminate social supports that are crucial to effective grieving.

By addressing their own mortality, a person may process their anxiety and fear (Yalom, 2009) and find meaning not only in the experienced loss, but also in their own lives. This may further enable adjustments that are needed to progress after loss, potentially paving the way for forming new, healthy life goals.

GOAL

This process addresses the 3rd and 4th Task of Mourning. It facilitates the exploration of existential questions and mortality. It provides those who are grieving an opportunity to process any fears or anxieties they may be feeling, eventually allowing for future goal setting and life planning.

MATERIALS

Paper or canvas	Crayons
Paint	Magazine/book clippings
Markers/pens	Scissors
Color pencils	Glue
Pastels	Clay/Model Magic

INSTRUCTION

Ask the client to consider any thoughts or feelings they have had around their own mortality. How do they view their life in the context of being mortal? What questions about life and death have come up for them since their loss? When they are ready, ask them to create an image that represents their view of their own mortality.

POSSIBLE PROCESSING QUESTIONS AND PROMPTS

After your client completes their piece, ask them to reflect on their creation and consider the thoughts and feelings they have identified. The following questions may be used to further explore the process.

1. Can you tell me about your piece and how it represents your feelings about your own mortality?

2. How do you think your experiences with loss have impacted your feelings about your mortality? About life in general?

3. How did it feel to consider your own mortality?

4. When you considered your mortality did you notice any emotions or physical sensations?

5. If you could assign one emotion word to your piece, what would it be? What does this word mean to you?

6. Do you feel like your views on your own mortality are impacting your life? If so, how?

7. Are there any elements that you would like to change about your views on mortality? How could you accomplish this change?

8. How do you think changing your view of your own mortality would impact your life? Your grief?

9. Do you think your feelings about your mortality have impacted your views of the future? How so?

10. How do you give your life meaning? How does this meaning impact your functioning? Your grief? Your future goals?

WHAT COMES AFTER?

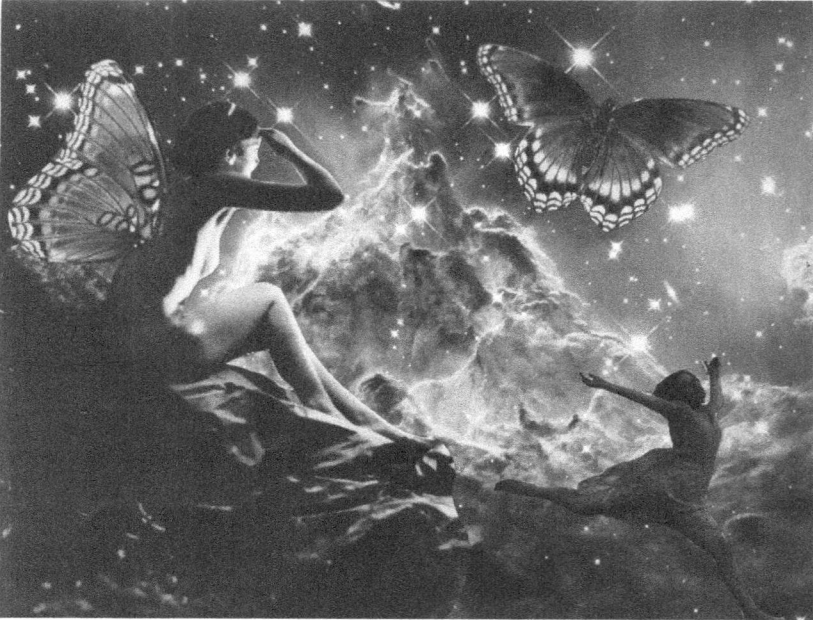

Figure 33: What Comes After?

PURPOSE

Worden (2018) noted that spiritual adjustments are critical for the 3rd Task of Mourning. He observed that a person must "attempt to reconstruct a world of meaning that has been challenged by the loss" (p.49). Without these adjustments a person may be at risk for complicated spiritual grief, including such reactions as changes in spiritual beliefs, even anger toward God.

One critical component of a person's spiritual beliefs is how they conceptualize what may occur after death (Worden, 2018), a drive that harks back to our earliest human ancestors in their attempt to remain hopeful for the deceased and alleviate their own death anxiety (Servaty-Seib & Chapple, 2021). Of course, such views on an afterlife vary between clients, depending on their cultural and spiritual beliefs. These may range from someone who is an atheist maintaining that there is nothing to someone who is Christian believing in heaven. What a person believes may impact how they grieve. For example, if a person believes in heaven, they may find peace that their loved one is with God in such a beautiful place. However, on the flip side, this person may also fear that the soul of their loved one has been sent to hell for an eternity of punishment. As comforting as heaven may be, the concept of hell may be equally terrifying and distressing.

Regardless of their beliefs, spiritual adjustments are necessary for effective grief counseling (Worden, 2018). By exploring them, a person may be able to accept the reality of the death while still recognizing the impact that their spiritual beliefs have on accepting or adjusting to their loss.

GOAL

This process addresses the 1st and 3rd Task of Mourning. Its focus is to help the client examine their beliefs about what happens to a person after they die, and how it impacts their own acceptance and adjustment to such loss, including the positive and negative impacts of their beliefs.

MATERIALS

Paper or canvas

Paint

Markers/pens

Color pencils

Pastels

Crayons

Magazine/book clippings

Scissors

Glue

Clay/Model Magic

INSTRUCTION

Ask the client to take a few moments to consider what their personal beliefs are about what happens to a person after they die. Where does the person/soul go after death? How do they feel these beliefs are impacting their grief? When they are ready, ask them to create a piece depicting their beliefs and views of what happens to a person after death.

POSSIBLE PROCESSING QUESTIONS AND PROMPTS

After your client completes their piece, ask them to reflect on their creation, focusing on how it reflects their beliefs. The following questions may be used to further explore the process.

1. Can you tell me about the piece you have created?

2. Can you share with me your belief on what happens when we die?

3. How is that depicted in your creation?

4. If you could assign one word to describe your artwork, what would it be? What does that word mean to you?

5. How do you feel when you look at this piece?

6. How do you feel these beliefs impact your grief?

7. How do you think these beliefs impact your life in general?

8. Can you think of any specific times where your beliefs were helpful in your grief journey? Harmful? How so?

9. Are there any changes you would like to make around your beliefs and their impact on your grief? What steps could you take to make these changes a reality?

CONNECTING TO THE DIVINE

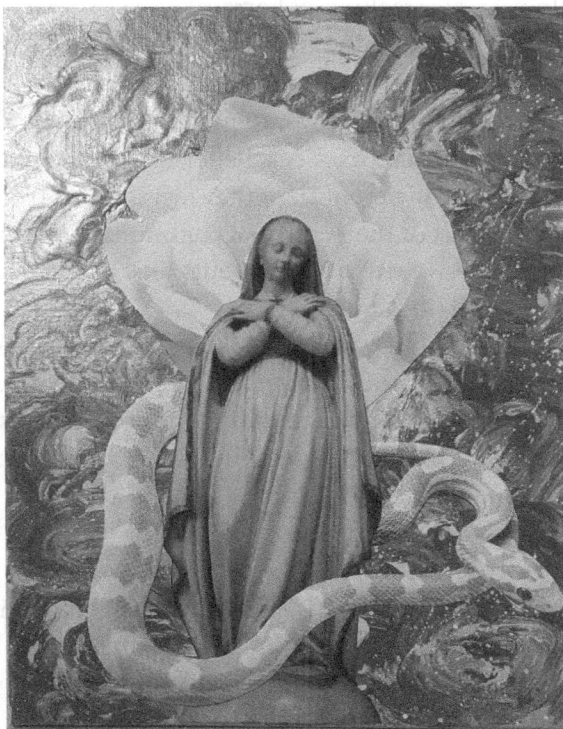

Figure 34: Connecting to the Divine

PURPOSE

The radical change associated with loss often brings a spiritual crisis (Doka, 2002; Worden, 2018). This is especially true in cases of sudden or unexpected loss, and for those who have strong religious or spiritual beliefs. A person may find themselves feeling angry towards a god they felt betrayed them. They may become bitter as they begin to mistrust the religion that was once a source of comfort.

These emotions may become feelings of disenfranchisement if the religious community they once relied on for sources of comfort during times of need fails to provide it for them (Doka, 2002). For example, a woman who was deeply religious and an active member of her church lost her mother with whom she shared a close connection. Although she always prepared food deliveries for other bereaved church members, she found that members of her church did not do the same for her. She began to question the true goodness of God and His followers. Her feelings of betrayal were so great she chose to leave her church of 15 years to find one that was more aligned with her principles, thus experiencing a new loss to grieve.

To help a person fully adjust to their loss, they must also address and adjust their spiritual practices, beliefs, and expectations. They may need to process any resentment they feel towards God, unhappiness with the support of their spiritual community, and any changes in their own beliefs. Spiritual adjustments may be a critical element to a person's overall life adjustments.

By encouraging a client to explore their spiritual beliefs, they may be able to process any associated and unexpected negative emotions and disappointments to begin rebuilding the connections with their faith. This may aid in meaning making, increased hope, and may protect against complicated grief.

GOAL

This process addresses the 3rd Task of Mourning. It facilitates a client's exploration of their connection to spiritual/religious beliefs and how these beliefs may impact their grief. It allows for the processing of emotions and goal formation related to fulfilling any unmet spiritual needs. It may further facilitate meaning making.

MATERIALS

Paper or canvas	Crayons
Paint	Magazine/book clippings
Markers/pens	Scissors
Color pencils	Glue
Pastels	Clay/Model Magic

INSTRUCTION

Ask the client to consider their religious/spiritual beliefs and what role these beliefs play in their lives. How have their spiritual beliefs changed after their loss? When they are ready, ask the client to create a piece that represents the impact of religion/spirituality in their lives and grief.

POSSIBLE PROCESSING QUESTIONS AND PROMPTS

After your client completes their piece, ask them to reflect on what they created. The following questions may be used to further explore the process.

1. Can you tell me about your piece and the beliefs you have chosen to depict?

2. What role did your spiritual beliefs play in your life before your loss? After?

3. How do you think your beliefs have shaped you as a person?

4. What emotional needs do your beliefs meet? How do your beliefs meet these needs?

5. What meaning do your beliefs give to death? To grief?

6. How does this meaning impact you and your grieving process?

7. How do you currently engage with your spirituality? Has this changed since your loss? If so, how?

8. Are you happy with the current role spirituality plays in your life? Would you like to see the role increased? Decreased?

9. What steps could you take in the future to meet your spiritual/religious needs?

PATH OF INITIATION

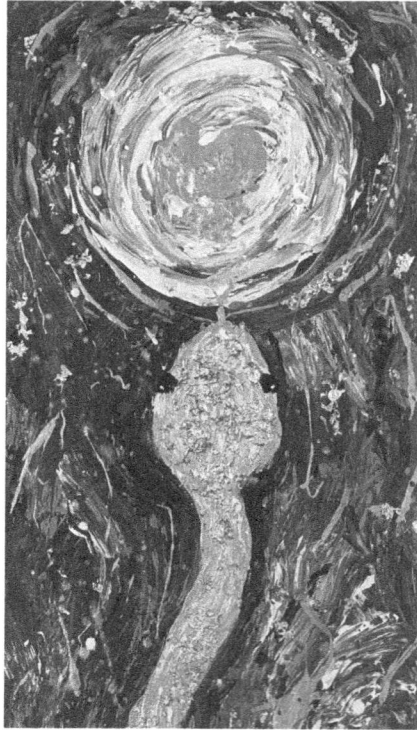

Figure 35: Path of Initiation

PURPOSE

A person's life is filled with transitions often marked by initiation rituals that they may not even be aware of (Moore & Havlick, 2001). Examples of commonplace initiation rituals include baptisms, birthdays, weddings, and graduations—events that mark personal evolution and life transitions.

While we may view many of these transitions and initiations as joyous, some may also contain an element of grief as a person moves from one phase of their life and identity into another (Moore & Havlick, 2001). As with all grief, the intensity will often directly relate to how attached a person was to the former phase of life. For example, an individual may feel excited to marry their partner, but also grieve the loss of their single lifestyle. Or a recent graduate may look forward to a career while also feeling sad, longing for the structure and friendships of college life.

Many life transitions require a certain degree of re-acclimation and reorganization (Moore & Havlick, 2001). This includes death, which, as an initiation, takes the bereaved from one phase of life into a new and uncertain one. During their grief they may feel they are living in a liminal space where the lives they experienced before the death and the life after the death collide. Grieving effectively helps the person continue through this liminal space and fully engage in the new phase of their lives.

All initiation rituals are used to mark these major life changes and help the transition from one phase into another with new knowledge and insight (Moore & Havlick, 2001). If the bereaved views their loss also as an initiation, it may aid their transition through grief and its uncertainty of the future. It may allow them to find meaning in the loss and facilitate effective grieving.

GOAL

This process addresses the 3rd and 4th Task of Mourning by asking the client to consider the idea of grief as a path of initiation. Its focus is to raise awareness of the greater life-changing impact of their grief and the possibility for growth and positive life change. It allows for possible goal setting that may increase self-efficacy, meaning making, and mastery.

MATERIALS

Paper or canvas	Crayons
Paint	Magazine/book clippings
Markers/pens	Scissors
Color pencils	Glue
Pastels	Clay/Model Magic

INSTRUCTION

Ask the client to take a moment to consider the idea of grief as an initiation or rite of passage. Ask them to consider other times in their lives that have felt they have gone through great life changes. Common ones could be puberty, marriage, divorce, birth of a child, etc. Then ask them to consider their loss and grief. How is their current grieving journey like an initiation? When they are ready, ask them to create a piece around the idea of initiation. This piece could reflect where they are currently on this path, their general view of the concept, or their feelings about being initiated into a new life by grief.

POSSIBLE PROCESSING QUESTIONS AND PROMPTS

After your client completes their piece, ask them to take time to reflect on their creation. The following questions may be used to further explore the process.

1. Can you tell me about your piece and how it shows your ideas of being initiated by grief?

2. What are your thoughts on the idea of grief being a rite of passage or an initiation? Had you considered your grief in this way before?

3. How did it feel to view your grief as a whole experience as opposed to each individual emotion and struggle?

4. Do you think considering grief as an initiation has changed your views about the grieving process? How so?

5. How do you feel your loss has changed you as a person? How do these changes compare with previous times you have experienced great change or rites of passage?

6. What do you hope to gain from this process of initiation? What changes do you hope to see in yourself?

7. What are some actions you feel you could take to help create this hoped-for change?

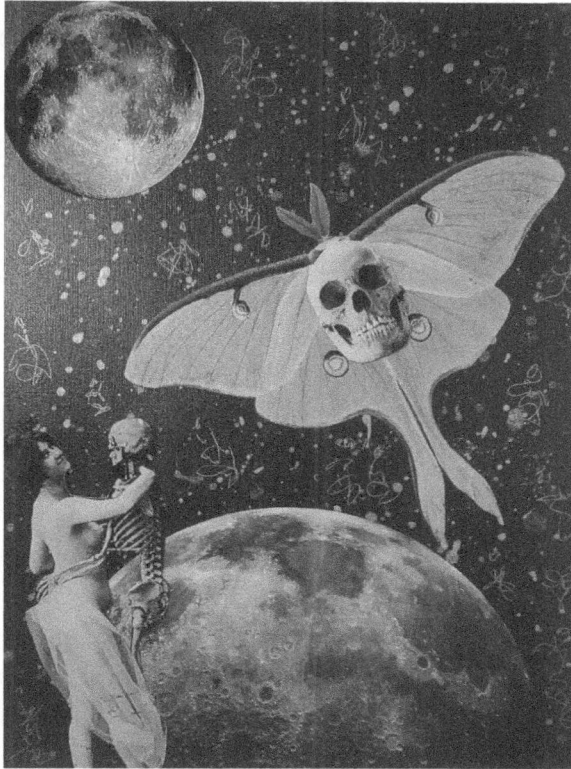

Figure 36: Transformation

PURPOSE

Loss, by its very nature, creates change. Such changes range from minorly inconvenient to life-altering (Doka, 2002). Of course, loss that creates the greatest change and upheaval in a person's life results in heightened feelings of grief. For a person to effectively grieve they must adjust to these radical life changes (Worden, 2018).

Meaning making after loss has emerged as one of the critical issues in grief work (Thompson & Neimeyer, 2014). Loss can challenge a person's beliefs about their lives, which, when unaddressed, may result in complicated grief. The meaning assigned to the loss event will depend on the individual and their beliefs, but finding meaning or purpose in a loss may help a person conceptualize the loss as beneficial—even if it is destructive—thus increasing feelings of hope and self-efficacy.

One way to help a client find meaning after loss is to explore the opportunity for personal transformation (Taylor, 2021). Transformational thinking may help a person change the focus of the grief from the devastation of loss to the hope for the future. By asking themselves how they might harness the experiences loss has forced upon them, they may be able to explore their own personal journey. The person they were prior to the loss is gone, but they have power in creating who they will become. The loss is no longer solely an event that happened to them but becomes an opportunity for inner reflection and personal change.

Exploring the transformational elements of grief may empower the individual to make healthy and beneficial changes in their lives by adding a new layer of meaning to their loss and the impact it has had on them.

GOAL

This process addresses the 3rd and 4th Task of Mourning by asking the client to consider their journey through grief and how this journey will transform them. It strives to aid in meaning making and increasing feelings of self-efficacy and control. It allows for the opportunity for goal formation related to their hoped-for transformation and ways to increasing feelings of self-efficacy.

MATERIALS

Paper or canvas	Crayons
Paint	Magazine/book clippings
Markers/pens	Scissors
Color pencils	Glue
Pastels	Clay/Model Magic

INSTRUCTION

Ask the client to consider how their grief has changed them and continues to change their lives. Ask them to consider the idea of transformation. A visual representation of this could be the caterpillar transforming into a butterfly. What does it mean to transform? When they are ready, ask them to create an image of their hoped-for transformation.

POSSIBLE PROCESSING QUESTIONS AND PROMPTS

After your client completes their piece, ask them to reflect on their creation and consider their journey and potential for positive change. The following questions may be used to further explore the process.

1. Can you tell me about your piece and the transformations you have chosen to show?

2. What does it mean to you to transform?

3. Can you think of other times in your life that you would describe as transformational? How did the transformation impact you?

4. How did it feel to look at your grief as a journey of transformation?

5. Prior to this exercise, had you considered the possibility of creating positive changes through your grief journey?

6. How did it feel to consider the changes you hope to see from this journey?

7. Do you think you are on the path to reach your hoped-for transformations? How so?

8. If you are not on the path to your hoped-for changes, what do you think you could do to create these changes?

FINGER LABYRINTH

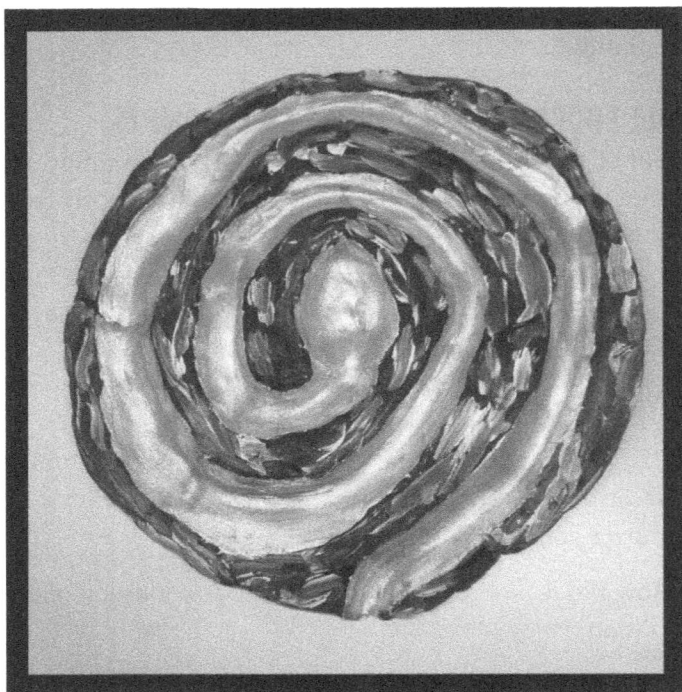

Figure 37: Finger Labyrinth

PURPOSE

The labyrinth has been used a spiritual tool for reflection and intro-spection since early human history (Plugg & McCormick, 1997). Tra-ditionally a large circular path spiraling towards a central circle and then spiraling back to the entrance, they were meant to be walked while in quiet contemplation of life and the journey of the soul. Unlike a maze, the labyrinth is not a puzzle to be solved, but a path to be followed.

In modern times, labyrinths have been used for many reasons, including as a tool to help the one walking the path reconnect with spirit and meditation (Plugg & McCormick, 1997). Creating and using labyrinths have also sparked interest and research in the field of psychology as it can be used for inner reflection and problem-solving, providing the opportunity to reflect on upon possible solutions (Peel, 2004).

The labyrinth has been adapted by some, taking them from large circles that are meant to be walked to smaller items typically created from clay that are only large enough for a finger to trace (Harris, 2002). Such finger labyrinths are more functional and accessible than the traditional labyrinths, particularly for those who may have space or ability limitations.

Commonly, the grieving individual will report feeling outside of their body or feeling disconnected from the world around them (Worden, 2018). By creating labyrinths from clay there is the benefit of using a material that often facilitates grounding while returning a sense of structure to the client (Hinz, 2020).

In grief work, the labyrinth may become a valuable tool to encourage mindfulness, introspection, and future planning. Creating the finger labyrinth, and any subsequent embellishments or decorations, may reinforce the uniqueness of the client's grief while also becoming a tool for self-soothing and grounding. It may help them feel a sense of power over personal transformation.

GOAL

This process may address the 3rd and 4th Task of Mourning. Its focus is to help clients assess where they are on their transformational journey after loss and create a tool to facilitate grounding. It further provides an opportunity for future self-soothing and developing effective grounding techniques.

MATERIALS

Air dry clay   Paint

Sculpting tools

INSTRUCTION

Ask the client to take a moment to consider their grief as a journey to new self-discovery and growth. Discuss the difference between a maze that is a puzzle to solve versus a labyrinth, which is more of a directed journey to an internal destination and a return. Instruct clients to create a labyrinth in whatever size and shape feels right for them with the clay provided. Ask them to ensure that the path through the labyrinth is wide enough to allow their finger to smoothly follow it. Once the piece is dry, ask the client to paint/decorate their creation in a way they find meaningful and pleasing.

POSSIBLE PROCESSING QUESTIONS AND PROMPTS

After your client completes their labyrinth, ask them to take time to reflect on their creation and encourage them to take a few minutes, close their eyes, and trace the labyrinth. The following questions may be used to further explore the process.

1. If the labyrinth is viewed as a journey into oneself to come out anew, where do you see yourself on this journey? Are you going in or are you working your way back out?

2. How will you know when you have completed your transformation? What does that look like?

3. How does it feel to consider your grief as a transformative journey?

4. Can you think of another time in your life where outer struggle created inner transformation? What did you do to create that change? How is it similar to or different from your current grief journey?

5. What do you think you still need to do to fully transform?

6. How did it feel to create the labyrinth? Did you notice any changes in your mood or body?

7. How did it feel to trace the labyrinth? How did your mood/body change?

8. Do you think the labyrinth you have created might be useful in your grieving journey? How so?

MEDITATION CREATION

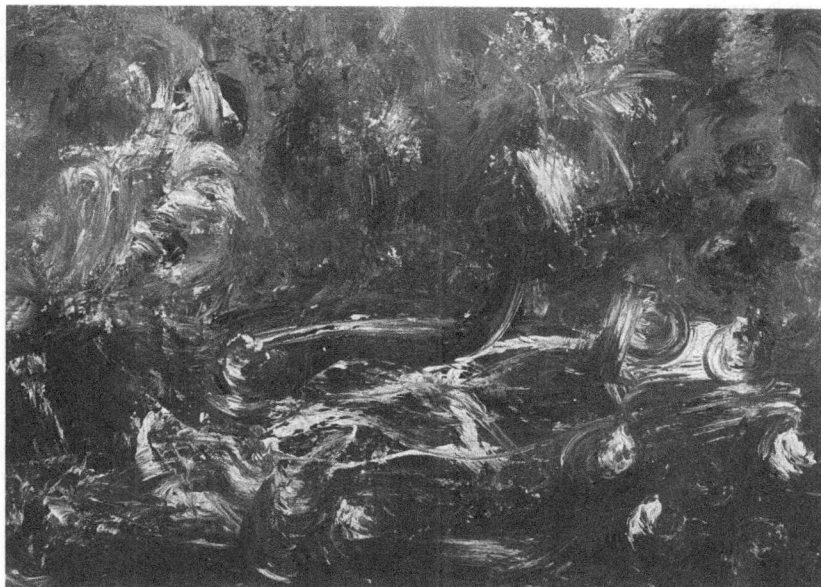

Figure 38: Meditation Creation

PURPOSE

Meditation has been used effectively in therapeutic practice to increase mindfulness and lower anxiety (Sagula & Rice, 2004). The study conducted by Sagula and Rice (2004) explored the impact of meditation on those experiencing chronic pain and grief due to an illness. They found that the group who engaged in meditation practices reported reduced depression and anxiety. They further found that the meditation group also advanced more quickly through their initial grief when compared to the control group.

Others have explored meditation as a tool not only for mindfulness, but also for healthy visualization (Doka, 2014). In such cases, it was used to aid the people who were ill with visualizing continued health, which helped them feel empowered and hopeful. It also aided in relaxation and general stress reduction.

Meditation may be either guided or unguided (Sagula & Rice, 2004). In guided meditation the client is read or listens to a relaxing story where they are typically asked to visualize things such as being in a peaceful location or seeing themselves filled with healing energy. In these cases, the client must only relax and visualize the scene they are hearing.

An alternative is the unguided meditation where a client is simply asked to sit quietly and let their mind wander without becoming too fixated on any one topic. They may be given a variety of visualizations to use if they begin to become focused on any one thought or emotion. In the unguided scenario, the individual has a measure of control with releasing their thoughts. This method of learning to release unwelcome thoughts or feelings may be a beneficial tool for intrusive thoughts or overwhelming emotions.

By employing unguided meditation and encouraging discussion on the thoughts or images that occurred, a person may gain new insight into their grief and their own healing needs, allowing for improved hope and possible goal formation.

GOAL

This process addresses the 3rd and 4th Task of Mourning. By facilitating a client's relaxed free thought through unguided mediation, new insight into their grief and needs may be gained. It may further add to stress-reducing tools and allow for goal setting related to self-care and grounding practices.

MATERIALS

Paper or canvas	Crayons
Paint	Magazine/book clippings
Markers/pens	Scissors
Color pencils	Glue
Pastels	Clay/Model Magic

INSTRUCTION

*Before the session, prepare an audio clip intended for unguided meditation.

Ask the client to sit in a comfortable position and close their eyes. Explain that you will spend five minutes sitting quietly listening to a unguided meditation/musical recording. Explain that they only need to sit and be present for the duration of the recording. Ask that they note where their mind goes during this time without becoming fixated on any specific thought. If a thought begins to overtake them, ask that they visualize the thought leaving them in a manner they find pleasing.

At the end of the time, ask the client to consider how the experience felt and consider any thoughts they had during the meditation. Ask them to create an image that depicts either their experience of sitting in meditation or any images that they saw in the meditation.

POSSIBLE PROCESSING QUESTIONS AND PROMPTS

After your client completes their piece, ask them to reflect on what they created and consider the time they spent in "stillness." The following questions may be used to further explore the process.

1. Can you tell me about your image? What element of the meditation experience does it depict?

2. How did it feel to take time to simply sit in stillness?

3. Did you notice any emotional or physical changes from before the meditation to after? What did you notice increasing? Decreasing?

4. What do you think the image you created is trying to tell you?

5. If you could assign one word to the image what would it be? The meditation? What do these words mean to you?

6. Was there anything about this experience or your image that stuck out to you? Why?

7. What is your overall impression of meditating in a free manner?

8. Do you feel adding a regular meditation to your life would be beneficial? How do you think it might change your feelings of anxiety, distress, anger, etc?

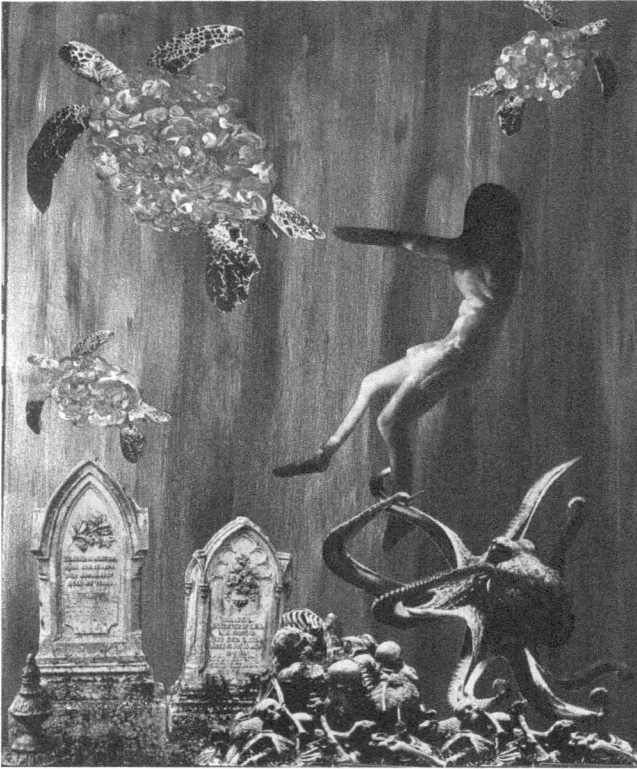

Figure 39: Where Am I Today?

PURPOSE

Grief is often a long, difficult journey that may consume a person's life (Worden, 2018). A person may become overwhelmed by what they believe is never-ending grief, unable to see any progress they have made. If a person becomes too overwhelmed, they may begin to withdraw. They may begin to engage in avoidant behaviors, such as working to excess or increasing substance use or alcohol consumption. These actions may devolve into a complicated grief process.

One way to address this overwhelming process is to check in

with the bereaved and explore where they feel they are in the here-and-now (Worden, 2018). Encouraging a person to put their grief on hold for a moment and focus on themselves may aid in changing their perspectives on their progress and current functioning. It may provide them the opportunity to see that they have indeed made important changes in their lives, thus increasing self-efficacy and hope.

This check-in may be done at various points during the therapeutic trajectory. By completing this suggested process at the beginning of therapy and then intermittently throughout, the changes the person may have made become more visible. This may encourage them to feel content or proud of the progress they have made and may motivate them to continue their grief journey with much more optimism and vigor.

Checking in also allows for a review and consideration of treatment goals, progress towards these goals, and any adjustments that may need to be made. By evaluating their goals, a person may increase their power and hope as they as they create new, or adjust existing, therapeutic goals.

GOAL

The process may address the 4th Task of Mourning. It aims to help the client examine their current functioning and evaluation of progress toward identified goals.

MATERIALS

Paper or canvas	Crayons
Paint	Magazine/book clippings
Markers/pens	Scissors
Color pencils	Glue
Pastels	Clay/Model Magic

INSTRUCTION

Ask the client to take a few moments to consider where they are currently in their grieving process and their life as a whole. How do they feel they are functioning? How are they processing their grief? When they are ready, ask them to create a piece that expresses where they are in this moment.

POSSIBLE PROCESSING QUESTIONS AND PROMPTS

After your client completes their piece, ask them to reflect on their creation and consider how it represents where they are in this moment. The following questions may be used to further explore the process.

1. Can you tell me about the piece you have created? How does it reflect your current functioning?

2. If you had to sum up your feelings about your current functioning in one word, what would that word be? Why?

3. How would you describe where you are emotionally? What do you think is going well? What do you think could be going better?

4. How do you feel your grief has impacted you as a whole person?

5. How did it feel to focus on the whole picture of you instead of just one element? Did this change your perspective of yourself? Your grief? How or how not?

6. Are there any areas in your functioning and grieving that you would like to change going forward? What would these changes look like? What steps do you think you could take to create this change?

7. How do you feel about your current goals? Are there any you feel need to be changed or adjusted? Which ones and why? What would these changes look like?

WHAT FEEDS ME?

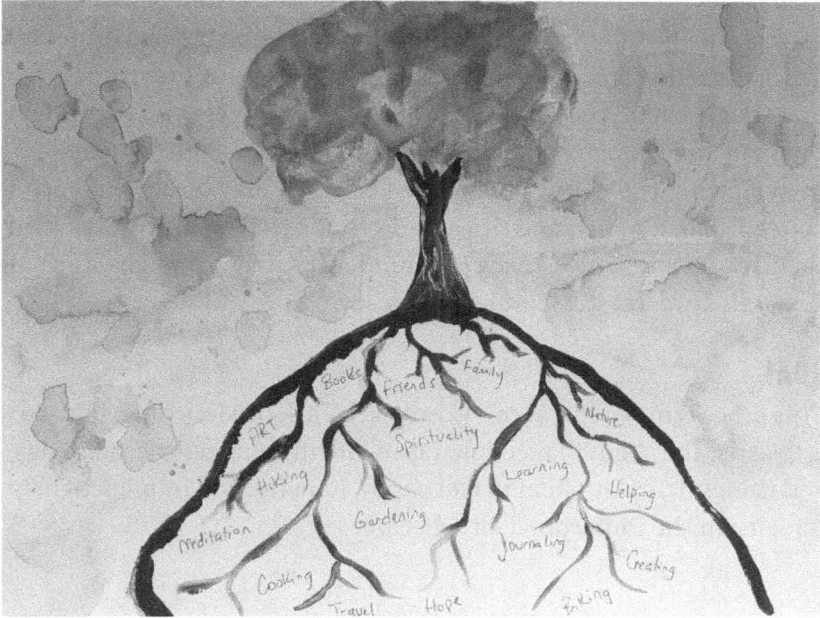

Figure 40: What Feeds Me?

PURPOSE

It is possible that after a loss and its subsequent grief journey a person loses touch with who they are and the things that made them feel good or whole (Worden, 2018). They may feel like their loss and grief has taken over their lives to such an extent that they no longer know who they are. They may stop engaging in activities they previously enjoyed. They may stop going to social events or withdraw from previous community groups. These actions may lead to increased isolation and depression. For example, an elderly widow stops going to church functions and lunch with friends, preferring to stay at home. She has stopped reading due to difficulty focusing and has discontinued her daily walks due to feeling tired. She finds herself spending endless hours thinking about her deceased husband and her increasing isolation and loneliness. This situation would put the client at an increased risk of complicated grief and potentially health consequences due to immobility (Worden, 2018).

Losing such connection with themselves may also make the Tasks of Mourning more difficult (Worden, 2018). If a bereaved person cuts themselves off from social support or disconnects from activities that increase feelings of control and mastery, they may have difficulty making needed life adjustments or setting goals for the future.

It may benefit a client to assist them in exploring who they are as a person and the activities and people that increase their happiness. By reviewing their lives before the loss, they may be able to better conceptualize which activities and groups they want to take into their future and which to leave behind. This may aid in goal formation, self-care, mastery, and self-efficacy.

GOAL

This process may address the 3rd and 4th Task of Mourning. Its focus is to assist the client in recognizing and identifying people, activities, and things that help them to feel happy, hopeful, and fulfilled to help refocus on the importance of self-care.

MATERIALS

Paper or canvas	Crayons
Paint	Magazine/book clippings
Markers/pens	Scissors
Color pencils	Glue
Pastels	Clay/Model Magic

INSTRUCTION

Ask the client to consider the things (activities, objects, people) in their lives that make them feel happy, fulfilled, hopeful, and inspired. What feeds their soul? When they are ready, ask them to create an image of a plant that represents themselves and below the plant, where the roots would be, ask them to list the things/people they have identified.

POSSIBLE PROCESSING QUESTIONS AND PROMPTS

After the client completes the piece, ask them to reflect on their creation and consider the people, activities, and things they have identified. The following questions may be used to further explore the process.

1. Can you tell me about the piece you have created and the things you feel feed you?

2. What is it about the plant you drew that you identify with? Was there a particular characteristic or feature that stuck out to you?

3. When you consider all the items you have listed, which do you currently engage in? Which have been put to the side?

4. How do you feel when you engage with these activities/people? Are these feelings different from how you are currently feeling?

5. Which person/activity listed has been the most helpful during times of struggle?

6. What identified people/activities do you feel you could give more energy or attention to?

7. Is there anything that you didn't list that you think might be helpful going forward?

8. What steps do you think you could take to help increase the time and energy you give to the areas you identified as creating positive feelings in your life? How do you think this might impact your grief? Daily functioning?

ANIMAL SYMBOL

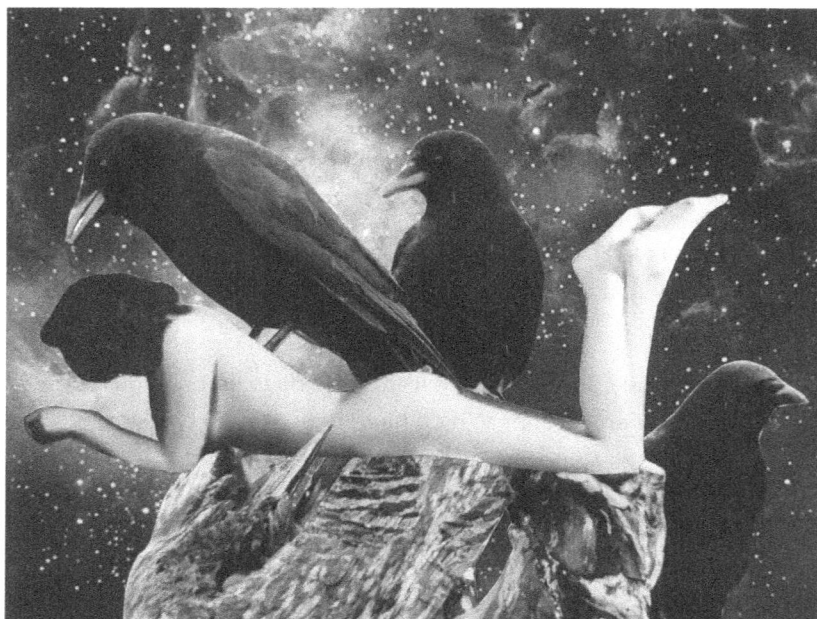

Figure 41: Animal Symbol

PURPOSE

When a person experiences a loss, they may be overcome by the emotions of grief (Worden, 2018). Some emotions, such as guilt or anger, may result in negative self-talk and self-abuse. If left unchecked, this will impact their self-esteem and self-image. For example, if a person is feeling guilty for their perceived responsibility in a loss, they may begin to believe they are an inherently bad person who deserves punishment. They may admit to feeling helpless in their ability to create the necessary change in their lives and ultimately feel hopeless for their future. If a person engages in negative self-talk or experiences lowered self-esteem, they may struggle to identify positive aspects of themselves (Kaduson, Schaefer, & Aronson, 2001). They may feel that they have no redeeming qualities and are unable to make positive changes in their lives. This mindset could block a healthy grieving process and ultimately impact their daily functioning. In such cases, it may be beneficial to help a person explore their strengths and how they could be reinforced to assist with their grief processing.

Positive attributes that a person struggles to identify in themselves may be more easily identified in others (Kaduson et al., 2001). One way to explore such necessary positive traits is to project such strengths onto an animal. Animals are often seen as embodying the human traits that a person most values or wishes to have. For example, people often see dogs as being loyal, birds as being free, or bears as being powerful. By asking a person to identify an animal they feel drawn to, they may be able to recognize why they chose that animals with its particular traits and eventually come to recognize these same qualities within themselves or explore how they could increase such characteristics within themselves. This may help improve self-efficacy, hope, self-esteem, and motivation, facilitating continuous healthy grieving and necessary life adjustments.

GOAL

This process may address the 2nd and 3rd Task of Mourning. It provides an opportunity for the client to identify current or desired strengths through the representation of an animal. It reinforces positive qualities and goal setting to increase identified desired traits and making needed life adjustments.

MATERIALS

Paper or canvas	Crayons
Paint	Magazine/book clippings
Markers/pens	Scissors
Color pencils	Glue
Pastels	Clay/Model Magic

INSTRUCTION

Ask the client to take a few moments to consider an animal that they admire or are generally drawn to. What draws them to this animal? How does the animal make them feel? When they are ready, ask them to create an image of their animal that highlights their identified traits and strengths.

POSSIBLE PROCESSING QUESTIONS AND PROMPTS

After your client completes their piece, ask them to reflect on their selected animal. The following questions may be used to further explore the process.

1. Can you tell me about your piece and what it represents?

2. Tell me about the animal you chose. Why did you pick this animal over all the others?

3. If you had to describe this animal in one word, what would it be? What does that word mean to you?

4. How does this animal make you feel?

5. What characteristics of this animal do you admire?

6. Are there any similarities between yourself and the animal you have chosen? What are they?

7. Are there any differences? What are they?

8. Are there any traits that this animal has that you wish you had? If so, what are they?

9. Do you think these traits would help you in your grief journey? How so?

10. What changes do you think you could make to help you acquire the traits you admire in this animal?

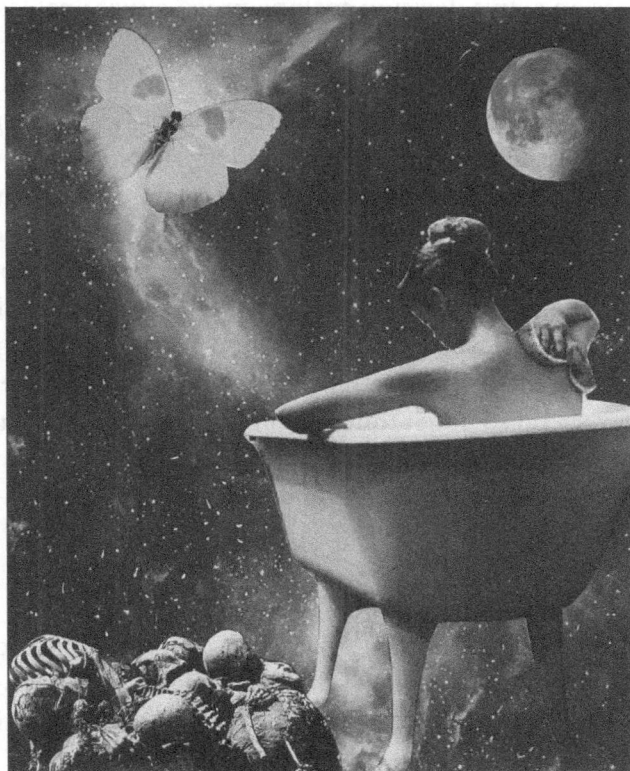

Figure 42: Caring for Me

PURPOSE

Self-care has seen increased attention in recent years, especially after the COVID-19 pandemic (Martinez et al., 2021). The need for such attention amid the responsibility to care for others became critical as new levels of emotional and physical burnout were experienced by healthcare workers during this time. Rates of complicated grief were expected to rise to levels never seen before (Gesi et al., 2020).

Self-care tends to be thought of as anything that generally

increases a person's sense of wellbeing. Martinez et al. (2021) attempted to formulate a more concrete definition. Through their study, they defined self-care as "the ability to care for oneself through awareness, self-control, and self-reliance in order to achieve, maintain, or promote optimal health and wellbeing [recognizing that] self-care is an active decision-making process that enables people to effectively engage in their care" (p.423).

Thus, it becomes apparent that self-care is necessary for effective grief work. Worden (2018) recognized that the greatest dangers to the bereaved are feelings of helplessness and hopelessness. By engaging in self-care activities that require decision making and focusing on the self, a person may experience increases in hope and self-efficacy.

Self-care may become particularly important when the bereaved are also caregivers. For example, if the widower is also a newly single father or if the bereaved is also a nurse or other caring profession. In such cases, the individual may have difficulty focusing on their needs when they spend so much time focusing on others (Worden, 2018). Exploring self-care activities or creating future self-care plans may help the bereaved reduce distress and increase feeling of self-efficacy and hope.

GOAL

The process may address the 4th Task of Mourning. Its focus is to help a client review any current self-care activities and allows for goal formation related to implementation of future self-care activities.

MATERIALS

Paper or canvas	Crayons
Paint	Magazine/book clippings
Markers/pens	Scissors
Color pencils	Glue
Pastels	Clay/Model Magic

INSTRUCTION

Ask the client to take a few moments to consider their current self-care habits or lack thereof. Ask them to consider how they feel before and after engaging in self-care. If they do not currently engage in self-care activities, ask them to consider how it might impact them to begin a self-care routine. When they are ready, ask them to create a piece that represents their self-care and its impact on them and their grieving journey.

POSSIBLE PROCESSING QUESTIONS AND PROMPTS

After your client completes their piece, ask them to reflect on their creation and consider their current self-care. Ask them to consider any changes in mood or body they felt when reflecting on taking care of themselves and creating their piece. The following questions may be used to further explore the process.

1. Can you tell me about your piece and how it represents your self-care?

2. If you were to rank your priorities, whether people or tasks, where would you rank caring for yourself? Has this changed due to your loss? If so, how?

3. Could you tell me about your current self-care routine? What do you like to do to care for yourself? How often are you engaging in this activity?

4. Have you noticed any differences in your mood before and after self-care activities? Any changes in your bodily sensations?

5. How do you feel your self-care practices have impacted your grieving?

6. If you do not currently have a self-care routine, how did it feel to consider starting one?

7. What activities that you are not currently doing do you feel would make you feel cared for? How do you think these activities would impact your grief?

8. What changes would you like to see in your self-care practice? What steps could you take to create these changes?

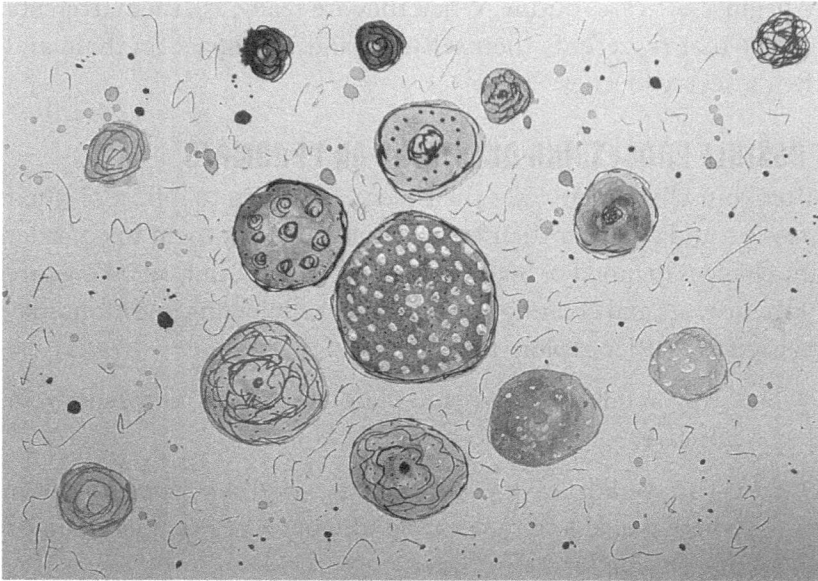

Figure 43: Circles of Support

PURPOSE

While grief is an individual experience, social systems serve several important functions in the grieving process (Doka, 2002). They provide a source of emotional support and comfort that assists with the first two Tasks of Mourning. They may also provide physical support, such as running errands or assisting with chores, aiding in the 3rd Task of Mourning. They may also serve as validation for an individual's grief, stemming off potential disenfranchisement.

It is normal during the early days of grief for a person to pull back from family and friends (Worden, 2018). Withdrawing from loved ones may occur as they feel unsupported, overwhelmed, or simply have a strong desire to be alone to process their loss. When someone experiences an intense grief response and engages in social isolation, they may have difficulty seeing the support systems available to them

(Worden, 2018). They may feel isolated and alone without realizing they have stopped accepting support from those around them. If gone unchecked, it may increase the likelihood of depression or complicated grief. Assisting a client to identify and reengage with the supportive friends, family, or groups in their lives may facilitate a successful grieving process and alleviate loneliness and isolation.

As already noted, however, with disenfranchised grief, social supports may be fewer (Doka, 2002). Helping the individual identify supports may be more difficult, but it is ultimately more critical as disenfranchised grief by its nature is isolative and essentially invisible. In such cases, it may be necessary to explore specialized support groups to create new and accepting systems.

GOAL

This process may address the 3rd Task of Mourning. Its focus is to identify your client's support systems and assess the strength of these supports. It also may help strengthen interpersonal relations.

MATERIALS

Paper or canvas	Crayons
Paint	Magazine/book clippings
Markers/pens	Scissors
Color pencils	Glue
Pastels	Clay/Model Magic

INSTRUCTION

Ask the client to reflect for a moment on the people in their lives. This can include family, friends, and organizations such as churches or support groups. Who in their lives has been helpful during previous difficulties? Who is helpful now? When they are ready, ask them to create a circle in the center of the paper provided to represent themselves. Next ask that they create additional circles to represent each person in their lives and how supportive they feel they are.

Ask that they place these circles in locations that show the person's level of support. For example, the most supportive people would be closest to the center and least supportive would be the farthest away. Encourage them to decorate each circle in a way that represents the individual/group.

POSSIBLE PROCESSING QUESTIONS AND PROMPTS

After your client completes their piece, ask them to reflect on their creation, particularly on the position and size of each circle. Ask them to consider how near or far the circles are placed to the circle representing themselves. The following questions may be used to further explore the process.

1. Can you tell me about the piece you have created and who is represented in each circle?

2. Who offers you the most support? Why do you see these people as the most supportive? What makes them supportive?

3. Who offers you the least support? Why do you view these people as least supportive? What makes them less supportive?

4. How comfortable are you reaching out to these individuals/ groups for support?

5. What encourages you to reach out for support? What discourages you from reaching out?

6. Does looking at this piece change the way you see your support system? If so, how?

7. Are there are individuals/groups that you would like to strengthen your bond with? If so, how can you accomplish this?

8. How would reaching out to support systems impact your grieving?

9. What steps can you take to become more engaged with the supportive people/groups in your life?

WHAT THEY SAID

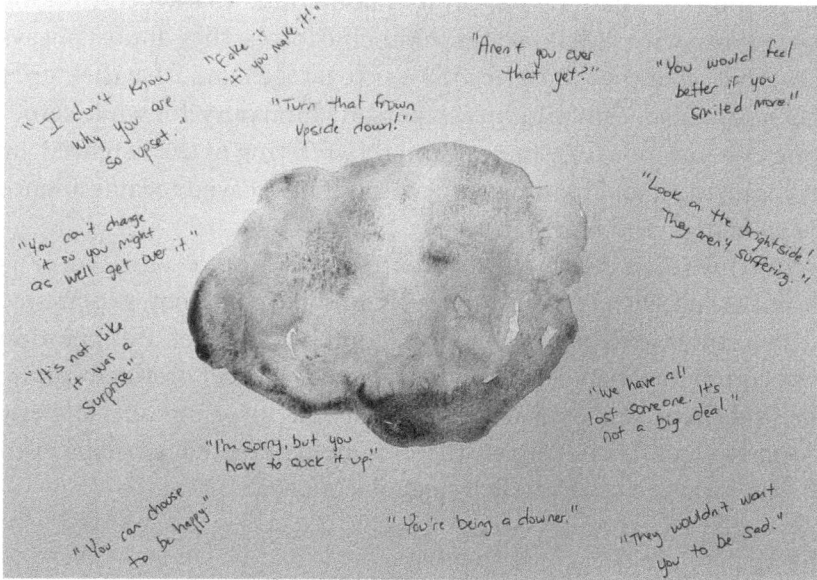

Figure 44: What They Said

PURPOSE

When people are faced with someone else's loss and grief, they often don't know what to do to show their love and support (Neimeyer, 2016). Combine this with people's natural inclination to fill the silence, a situation may arise where a well-meaning person may unintentionally say something that causes further hurt and confusion in the bereaved.

When confronted with loss, especially when the loss is sudden or traumatic, people feel the need to find meaning (Worden, 2018). This may result in statements that are meant to be comforting and supportive, but in fact compound the distress. For example, a recently widowed woman was told by a loved one "He is in a better place" and "God always has a plan for us." While this may have been meant to be comforting, the widow became angry and felt betrayed by God. In another example, a man who was diagnosed with cancer was told that he had gotten cancer because "God believed he was strong enough to beat it." Although an attempt to comment on his strength it only created anger and confusion.

What many well-meaning friends and family do not understand is that often what the bereaved need to hear most is simply "I am here and I see you" (Yalom, 2009). Yalom found that when working with those with illnesses or experiencing losses, they almost always said that what they most needed was to be seen and have their grief acknowledged. This reinforces a person's humanity, for while someone else may not truly understand the suffering of the bereaved, by recognizing it and holding space for it, the bereaved regains a sense of validation and acceptance.

Yet, when a person feels their grief is not recognized or is bombarded with well-meaning comments, they may experience disenfranchisement, evolving into complicated grief. By exploring the comments made to them, a person may reflect on the meaning behind them, process their emotional reactions, and alleviate any negative feelings or impact the comments created, perhaps even finding ways to counter their negative impact.

GOAL

This process may address the 2nd Task of Mourning. Asking the client to consider things that have been said to them about their loss and how it has impacted them may assist the client's ability to see these interactions more objectively and consider how a person's experiences may impact what they view as good advice. This, in turn, can empower the bereaved, granting them a sense of agency, allowing them to recognize where such statements derive from (i.e., the other's inability to find the right way to express their support or their sense of anxiety and discomfort in the face of another's loss) and, in turn, mitigate the negative reaction of the other's words. It further promotes work toward establishing future boundary setting and effective communication.

MATERIALS

Paper or canvas   Paint

Markers/pens	Pastels
Color Pencils	Crayons

INSTRUCTION

Ask the client to consider what others have said to them during their grieving process. What "advice" have those in their life given them to "help" them "get over" their grief? How has this impacted them? When they are ready, ask that they create a picture in the middle of the paper showing how these words have impacted them. Ask them to list around this image some of the words that have stuck out to them or impacted them the most.

POSSIBLE PROCESSING QUESTIONS AND PROMPTS

After your client completes their piece, ask them to reflect on the words they have written and the accompanying image. The following questions may be used to further explore the process.

1. Can you tell me about the image you created and how it shows the impact of others' words?

2. Can you share some of the words/sayings you have identified?

3. How have these impacted you and your grieving?

4. Are there any words you agree with? Disagree with?

5. How did you respond when these things were said to you? Did you communicate your feelings to the person saying them? Why or why not?

6. Did you notice any change in the relationship after the person shared their advice? If so, how did it change?

7. How do you feel about honestly communicating your feelings and needs with others? Why?

8. How do you think you could respond in the future when people say things about your grieving that you disagree with? How would this make you feel? Would it change the impact of what was said?

ENGAGING THE SENSES

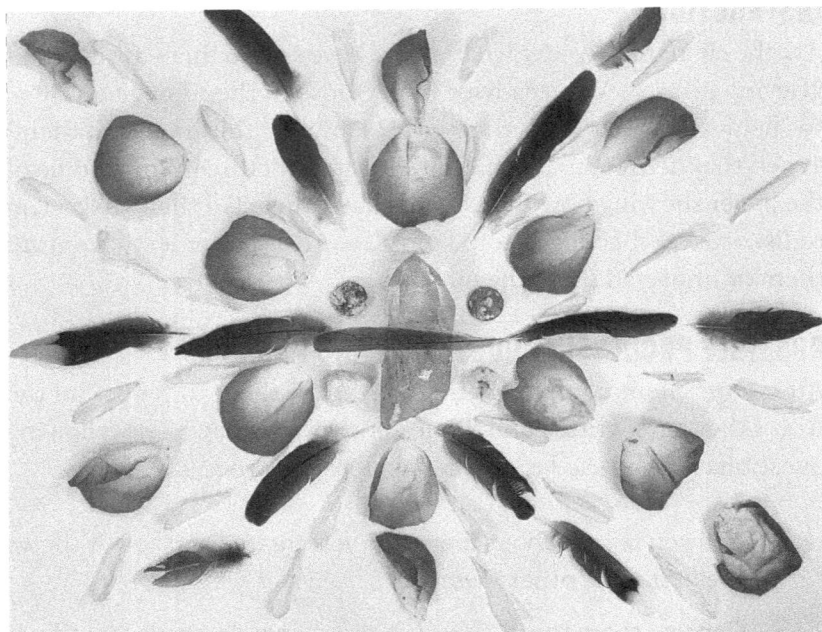

Figure 45: Sense Mandala

PURPOSE

After experiencing a loss, a person may report a variety of emotional and physical symptoms. They may indicate feeling disconnected and numb (Worden, 2018). They may experience disassociation, potentially creating barriers to the needs for daily living. For example, if an individual feels such disconnection or numbness, they may not recognize that they haven't eaten for some time, potentially devolving into extensive weight loss or disordered eating. They may develop a sleep disorder due to difficulty with relaxing.

People also report their thinking as fuzzy and unclear (Worden, 2018). Combined with feeling disconnected, this may create a situation where a person neglects their own needs and ability to act in a way consistent with their own best interests. When left unaddressed, this could create a negative spiral that becomes increasingly impactful on an individual's grief processing, eventually on their quality of life.

One way to address this is by helping them engage their senses (Neimeyer, 2012). By engaging the senses of touch, sight, and smell, a person may be able to return to the here-and-now and begin the process of reconnecting with their physical bodies, thoughts, and needs. Facilitating the reconnection with the body through stimulating the senses a person may become more aware of their own needs. This awareness may increase self-care behaviors and prevent unwanted physical consequences of grief. Such reconnections may, furthermore, decrease distress and anxiety.

GOAL

This process may address the 3rd Task of Mourning. Its focus is to help the client reconnect with their bodies by engaging their senses. It facilitates practicing mindfulness and reflection on feeling connected with themselves and their needs.

MATERIALS

Large white piece of paper   Sense-engaging objects

*This directive aims to engage the client's senses so you can also provide a variety of materials to stimulate different senses with varying textures, colors, and smells.

INSTRUCTION

Ask the client to take some time to engage with the materials you have provided. Ask them to hold them, smell them, notice their texture, color, and pattern. Ask that they take a few deep breaths and feel their bodies, becoming aware of being present in this space. When they are ready, ask them to create a mandala on the white paper using the materials provided. Ask the client to create slowly, purposefully, and while being present in the moment. Ask that they focus completely on the act of creation and, if any other thoughts come into their minds, to release the thought and bring their attention back to the materials in front of them. The objects should just be placed on the paper without gluing or taping to allow for movement and reuse. The creation of a piece that is not permanent can help the client engage more fully with the moment and reflect on the nature of life where only the present moment exists.

POSSIBLE PROCESSING QUESTIONS AND PROMPTS

After your client completes their piece, ask them to reflect on it and how they felt during its creation. The following questions may be used to further explore the process.

1. How did you feel before starting this exercise? What did you notice emotionally? Physically?

2. How do you feel now? What has changed?

3. How did it feel to consider the details of the objects you were working with?

4. How was this attention similar to or different from your everyday experiences?

5. Is there anything about your mandala that sticks out to you? If so, what? Why?

6. How did it feel to create slowly and with purpose? Did you notice any changes in your bodily sensations when you worked in this manner?

7. How do you think you can take this experience into your everyday life? How do you think this might change any feelings you have of disconnection?

NATURE WALK AND SCULPTURE

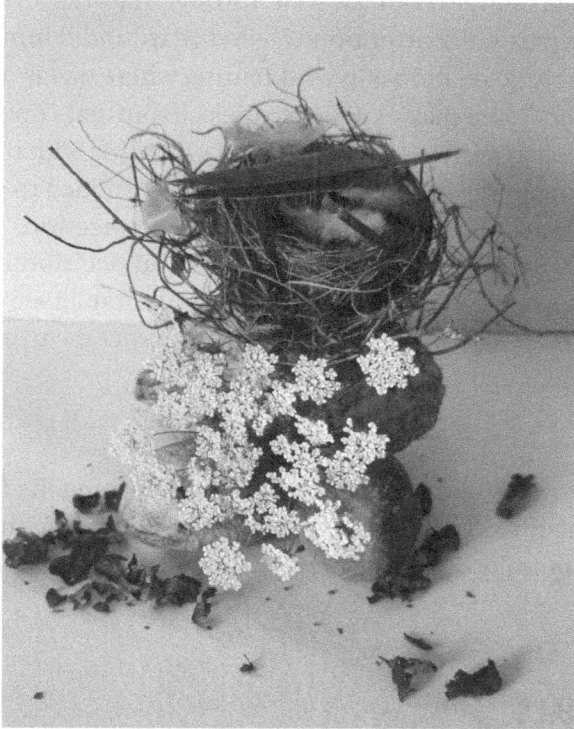

Figure 46: Nature Walk and Sculpture

PURPOSE

As underscored in the directive *Engaging the Senses*, it is common for the bereaved to experience feeling numb and disconnected from their physical bodies. This often leads to a variety of negative consequences, such as difficulty meeting their own needs (Worden, 2018). When left unaddressed, these feeling of disconnection and unmet needs could create barriers to effective grieving and begin to impact daily living.

Mindfulness exercises may aid in reconnecting with the physical body and increasing awareness of needs (Neimeyer, 2012). Helping the bereaved learn skills that can bring them from a place of thoughts and emotions to bodily awareness and presence may lower feelings of numbness and increase self-efficacy.

Mindfully engaging with nature may be a way for the bereaved to feel connected not only with themselves, but also with the world as a whole (Van Gordon, Shonin, & Richardson, 2018). This may be done through simply taking a walk through natural surroundings and paying particular attention to what is around. Humans often form a symbiotic relationship with nature, where one is dependent on the other. Some may experience deeper spiritual connection by mindfully engaging in nature and thus reconnecting with themselves.

Collecting items for later art creation can be added to the mindful nature walk, increasing awareness and connection. The focus of the individual shifts eventually to mindful decision making as items are selected based on appearance and desirability. By deciding which items are taken or left, the bereaved may come to experience empowerment and control.

GOAL

This process may address the 3rd Task of Mourning. Its focus is to help the client reconnect with their bodies by engaging their senses through mindfully collecting items from their environs and creating with them.

MATERIALS

Objects found in nature	Natural objects provided by therapist

INSTRUCTION

*Before this session ask the client to take a walk in a natural setting. This could be as simple as their own yard or a local park. Ask that they practice mindfulness when they are on their walk by being present in all aspects of their walk. They can accomplish this by noting the colors, smells, and sounds around them. Ask them to collect objects during their walk that they find interesting and that can be used for creation of a sculpture during session.

*Adjustments may be made to accommodate any limitations to walking in nature due to physical disability or location. You may also provide a variety of objects previously found in nature such as sticks, stones, feathers, etc.

Ask the client to take some time to engage with the materials that either they have collected or that you have provided. Ask them to hold them, smell them, notice their texture, color, and pattern. Ask that they take a few deep breaths and feel their bodies, becoming aware of being present in this space. When they are ready, ask them to create a sculpture representing connection with themselves using the materials they have selected.

POSSIBLE PROCESSING QUESTIONS AND PROMPTS

After your client completes their piece, ask them to reflect on what they have created and how they felt during its creation. The following questions may be used to further explore the process.

1. Can you tell me about the piece you have created?

2. Is there anything about your sculpture that sticks out to you? If so, what? Why?

3. How did you feel when you were walking in nature/selecting your materials? How were these feelings similar to or different from your everyday feelings?

4. What made you select the materials that you did? Do you notice any pattern in the materials you selected?

5. How did it feel to consider the details of the objects you were working with? How was this attention similar to or different from your everyday experiences?

6. How did you feel before starting this exercise? What did you notice emotionally? Physically? How do you feel now? What has changed?

7. How do you think you can take this experience into your everyday life? How do you think this might change any feelings you have of disconnection?

POWER

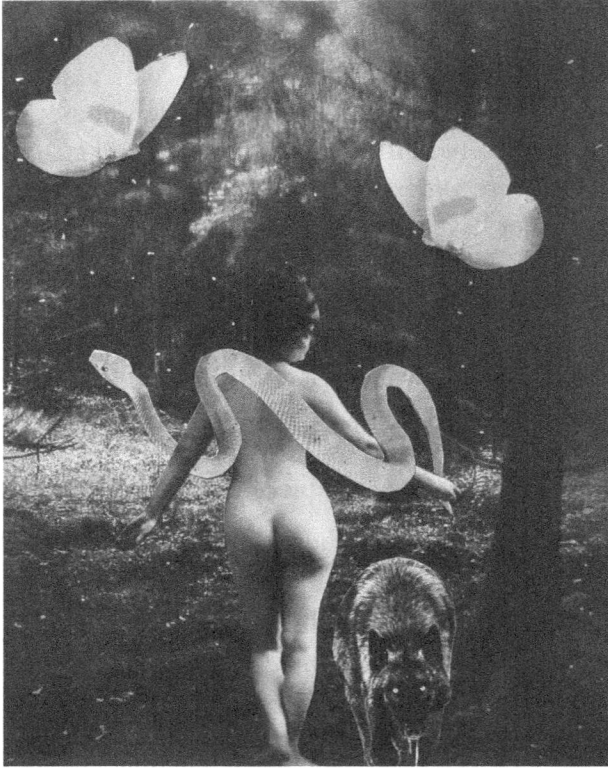

Figure 47: Power

PURPOSE

When and how a person experiences loss is often out of the person's control (Rando, 1984). While there are times when a person may facilitate or predict loss, such as a divorce or leaving a job, this is just as often not the case. Such lack of control can create a sense of powerlessness and helplessness (Worden, 2018). When left unaddressed these feelings may impact effective grief processing and the individual's future functioning.

To help a person increase a sense of control, it may be helpful to explore how the person perceives power (Rando, 1984). Just like grief, power will be conceptualized differently depending on the individual's personal beliefs and culture. For some, they may view power as the ability to control the outcome of a situation. Others may view true power as being able to relinquish control and adapt to change. For example, a person who has been diagnosed with cancer has little control over their treatments or the outcome of their disease, but they may come to realize they have the power to live and function in a way they choose despite their illness.

Regardless of how power is conceptualized, increasing one's sense of power may offset feelings of helplessness and improve grief outcomes (Worden, 2018). By exploring power and its meaning in one's life, the bereaved may be encouraged to take independent and beneficial actions in both their grieving and—ultimately—their lives.

GOAL

This process may address the 3rd Task of Mourning. By helping the client explore their thoughts around the meaning of power and where they have power in their own lives, it facilitates self-efficacy and mastery.

MATERIALS

Paper or canvas	Crayons
Paint	Magazine/book clippings
Markers/pens	Scissors
Color pencils	Glue
Pastels	Clay/Model Magic

INSTRUCTION

Ask the client to take some time to consider the idea of power. What is power? What does it feel like to have power or to be powerful? When they are ready, ask them to create a piece around the idea of power.

POSSIBLE PROCESSING QUESTIONS AND PROMPTS

After your client completes their piece, ask them to reflect on what they have created. The following questions may be used to further explore the process.

1. Can you tell me about your piece and how it represents your views on power?

2. What does the word power mean to you? What does it mean to be powerful or have power in your life?

3. What areas of your life make you feel powerful?

4. What areas of your life make you feel powerless?

5. What would it look like if you felt you had more power in your life? What would change?

6. How does your grieving make you feel powerless? Powerful?

7. How do you think feeling more powerful in your life would change your grieving?

8. What steps could you take to feel more powerful and in control of your life?

PAPER MOSAIC

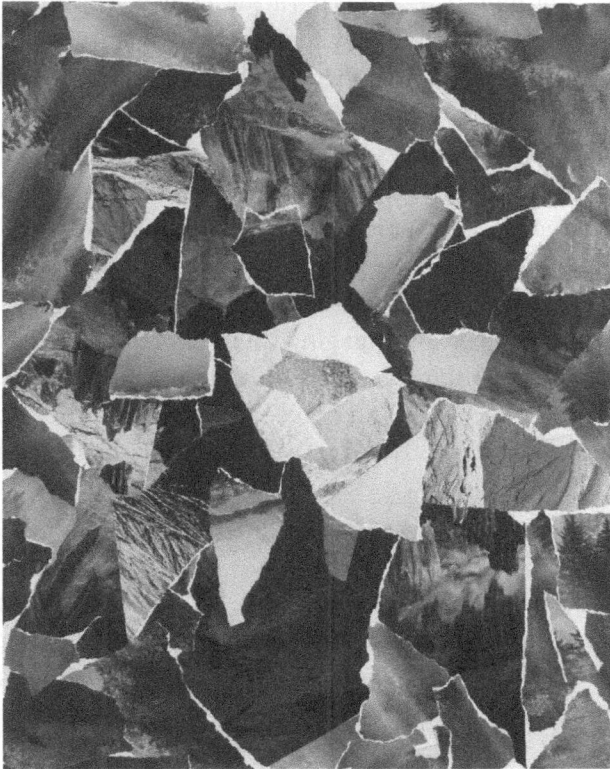

Figure 48: Paper Mosaic

PURPOSE

As discussed in the *Power* directive, loss and its impact on the life of the individual is often out of their control. When a person feels this way, they may begin to experience a loss of control over other areas of their lives (Worden, 2018). In more extreme cases, they may begin to adopt the belief that they are helpless and at the mercy of the destructive forces of life. As the helplessness increases, they may begin to feel hopeless and defeated. This could devolve into a self-fulfilling prophecy as they reinforce the patterns of inaction and withdrawal.

As part of the self-fulfilling prophecy, a person may begin to engage in maladaptive and destructive behaviors (Doka, 2002). These behaviors can range in their manifestations but usually share the common underlying themes of avoidance and control. When a person feels high levels of helplessness, they may experience a deep need to control something, even if it is harmful. They may even internalize the loss in such a way that they justify their harmful behaviors as deserved punishment for imagined transgressions, thus experiencing control as punisher and increasing helplessness as the punished.

There is a variety of ways to help someone reclaim their healthy feelings of control (Worden, 2018). One way is to engage them in the process of directed destruction and recreation. By channeling their destructive tendencies into controlled artistic expression, they may experience cathartic release and new perspectives on the control they have in their lives. By engaging them to create something new from the pieces of their destruction, they may see how they can begin to rebuild their lives and make meaning from their loss. This new meaning and perspective may help the individual increase their hope and self-efficacy.

GOAL

This process may address the 2nd and 3rd Task of Mourning. By helping the client to practice feeling in control and to gain perspective on the greater patterns of life, it encourages positive meaning making and hope.

MATERIALS

Blank paper   Colorful paper

Magazine pages   Glue

INSTRUCTION

Ask the client to select from five to ten images/pages that they find engaging and interesting. Discuss with the client how loss that is outside of their control can feel particularly destructive. Explain that this exercise it to allow them to symbolically reclaim their lost control. Then ask clients to spend one minute ripping the selected pages into pieces without considering size or shape. The goal is to just get lost in the act of ripping the pages. Next ask the client to create a new image using only the pieces of ripped pages and the materials provided. Ask them to refrain from any further ripping and limit their creation to only the pieces they have created.

POSSIBLE PROCESSING QUESTIONS AND PROMPTS

After your client completes their piece, ask them to reflect on what they created. The following questions may be used to further explore the process.

1. Can you tell me about the image you created and what it represents to you?

2. How did it feel to rip up the pages you selected? How is this feeling similar to the way you feel about your loss?

3. When you were ripping the pages what emotions did you experience? Sensations in your body?

4. How did it feel to create something new from the pieces of something that was destroyed?

5. Did you notice any changes in your emotions/body sensations between destruction and creation? How would you describe these changes?

6. How are you feeling now compared with before you started the project?

7. How in control of your life do you currently feel? What would help you feel more in control?

8. What would you like to create in your own life? What steps could you take to help make this change?

NEW ROLE

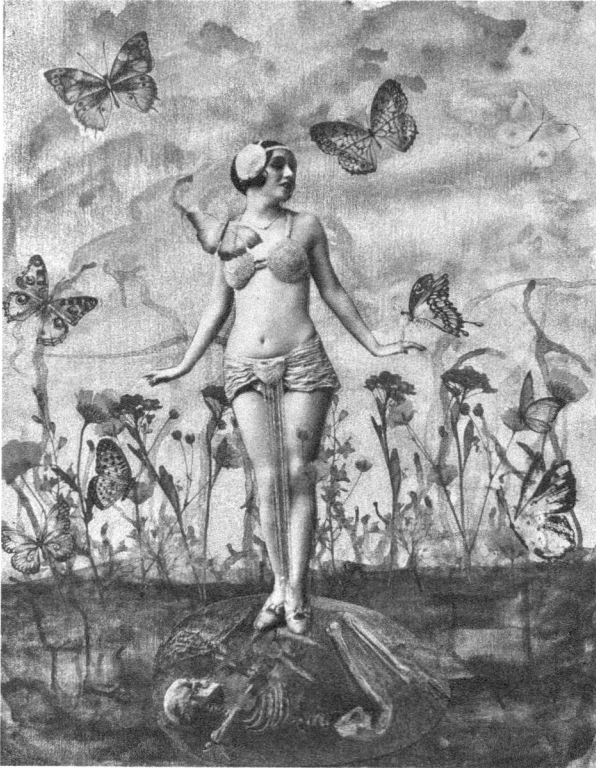

Figure 49: New Role

PURPOSE

Life and social interactions are a complex system of interconnecting roles (Worden, 2018). A woman may take on many roles, including wife, mother, professional, homemaker, daughter, and sister. Other members of a family are often assigned many other roles, including parent, child, financial provider, and caregiver. However, after a loss, these roles often need to be adjusted and adapted.

For example, if a woman had been the primary caregiver to her children, her death, or even a chronic and life-threatening illness that leaves her unable to fulfill the expected responsibilities of her role, will create a vacancy that will need to be filled by another. If a college student discovers they have cancer and can no longer continue with school, they have lost their socially granted identity of student and will find themselves adapting to a new role and identity.

Role adjustment is the focus of the 3rd Task of Mourning (Worden, 2018). A person who has experienced a loss that alters their life needs to make both large and small adjustments, taking on not only the new role, but also the various nuances and responsibilities of that identity. For example, a widow or widower not only has to adjust to the loss of a spouse, but must also complete all the spouse's typical activities, such as taking out the garbage, cooking, getting the mail, and paying the bills. If the bereaved person had been financially dependent on the one they have lost, they will have to adjust to the loss of income and how life will be altered because of decreased finances and a need to work more.

Such role adjustments are not only external, but internal as well. The bereaved must also adjust to their new identity: the wife becomes the widow, the healthy becomes the sick, the child becomes the orphan. Exploring the new role and new identity is essential for increasing control and hope. It may facilitate healthy problem-solving to meet the needed adjustments, ultimately increasing self-efficacy and mastery.

GOAL

This directive may address the 3rd Task of Mourning. It aims to facilitate the consideration of new roles and identities due to loss. It allows for problem-solving and goal setting related to the meeting the needs of their new role. It may increase hope, self-efficacy, and mastery.

MATERIALS

Paper or canvas	Color pencils
Paint	Pastels
Markers/pens	Crayons

| Magazine/book clippings | Glue |
| Scissors | Clay/Model Magic |

INSTRUCTION

Discuss with the client the various roles a person may assume in life. Ask them to consider what their role was before their loss and how that role has changed since their loss. What new needs must they meet? What new tasks must they perform? When they are ready, ask them to create a piece about the new role they fill and how they are feeling about the role.

POSSIBLE PROCESSING QUESTIONS AND PROMPTS

After your client completes their piece, ask them to reflect on what they created. The following questions may be used to further explore the process.

1. Can you tell me about your piece and the role it symbolizes?

2. What did your role look like before your loss? What role did the thing/person you lost play in your life?

3. What does your new role look like? How do these changes make you feel? Why?

4. What part of your new role do you find most difficult? Are there any things that make this role easier? What are they?

5. Are there any aspects of your new role you are struggling to meet? What would decrease this struggle?

6. What aspects of your new role have been successful? How has this success impacted you? Your grief?

7. Are there any aspects of your new role that you find rewarding or adding to your growth?

8. As you look toward the future, what areas of your new role still need to be addressed? What steps can you take to meet these future role needs?

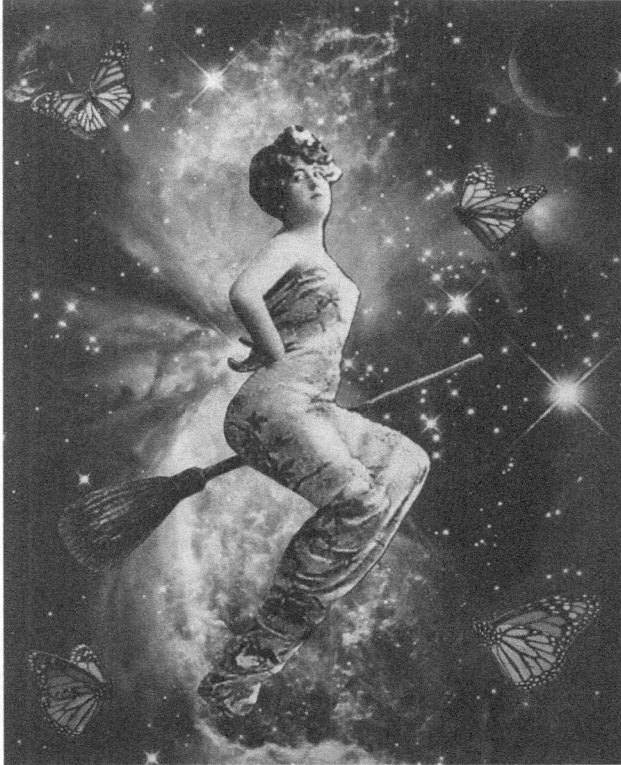

Figure 50: Hope

PURPOSE

Hope is critical for effective grieving and creating healthy life adjustments after loss (Worden, 2018). Contrariwise, hopelessness may increase feelings of longing, despair, and helplessness, as the person may view the world as cold and empty. They may feel that their futures are not worth fighting for if all they see in the foreseeable future is continuous suffering.

Hope has been considered necessary to facilitate adjustment to a variety of trauma and loss (Valle, Huebner, & Suldo, 2006). People who reported greater feelings of hope also reported lower levels of distress, despair, and sadness, and greater feelings of self-efficacy; they tended to take more positive actions and engage in productive behaviors (Valle et al., 2006).

Hope and effective coping strategies were shown to positively influence prognosis and survival in those with life-threatening and chronic illnesses (Doka, 2002). For example, a hopeful person is more likely to comply with treatment recommendations and engage in positive life changes to aid recovery and survival.

On the contrary, hopelessness may create a barrier to grieving and increase risk of complicated grief, sometimes leading to suicide (Latham & Prigerson, 2004). Instilling hope early in the grieving process may protect against such complicated grief and help offset the resultant suicidal ideation.

Loss creates the need for various life adjustments both internally and externally (Worden, 2018). Feeling hopeful may allow the person to more easily envision a new, desirable life after loss. Increasing feelings of hope may further improve coping, increase self-efficacy, and aid in meaning making.

GOAL

This process may address the 3rd and 4th Task of Mourning. Asking the client to explore their ideas of hope and what they hope for as they work with their grief and loss promotes goal formation that will assist in reaching their identified future desires. This may lead to self-efficacy and meaning making.

MATERIALS

Paper or canvas	Crayons
Paint	Magazine/book clippings
Markers/pens	Scissors
Color pencils	Glue
Pastels	Clay/Model Magic

INSTRUCTION

Ask the client to consider the idea of hope. What does it mean to have hope? How have their views of hope changed since their loss? What makes them feel hopeful? When they are ready, ask them to create a piece related to the idea of hope and what they hope for going forward.

POSSIBLE PROCESSING QUESTIONS AND PROMPTS

After your client completes their piece, ask them to reflect on their creation and consider their ideas of hope and their future life. The following questions may be used to further explore the process.

1. Can you tell me about your piece and how it reflects your ideas about hope? What element of hope have you represented?

2. Is there any part of your creation that stands out more than others? If so, why?

3. What does it mean to you to have hope or to be hopeful?

4. How do you think your feelings and behaviors change when you feel hopeful? Did you notice any changes in your feelings when you were considering hope and creating your piece?

5. Do you feel your own hope has changed since your loss? If so, how?

6. How hopeful do you feel for your future? What could increase your feelings of hope?

7. If you were to select one thing you hope for most in the future, what is it? Why did you select that particular thing?

8. What actions do you think you are currently taking to reach your hoped-for future? What steps do you think you could take?

VISION OF THE FUTURE

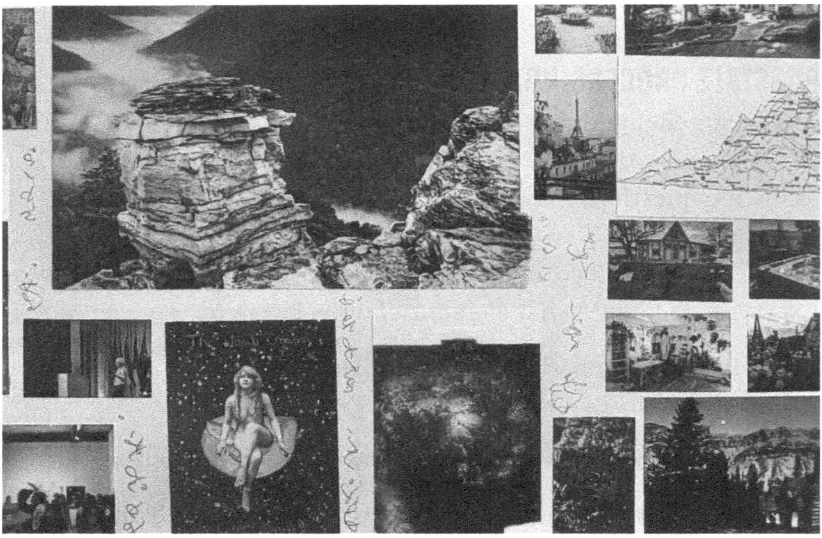

Figure 51: Vision of the Future

PURPOSE

The goals of grief counseling are multifaceted. It is not only accepting the loss and its emotional impact, but also how a person engages with life after loss. Successful reintegration afterwards includes an individual's ability to remember what was lost while still progressing into their new life (Worden, 2018). In other words, the bereaved successfully shifts from viewing the past and the loss's impact on their present life to their hoped-for future.

At first, the idea of a future after loss may seem overwhelming (Worden, 2018). The bereaved may struggle with identifying goals and aspirations due to the emotional or physical impact. If addressed too early in the therapeutic relationship and too soon after the loss, a person may be too numb to consider anything other than their presenting emotional state.

In cases where a client has difficulty engaging in visualizing their future or difficulty expressing what it might look like, creating a vision board may help (Burton & Lent, 2016), as it helps them form their thoughts or feelings into concrete expression. This may, in turn, instill hope and promote problem-solving, particularly on how to achieve their goals. It turns their discombobulated, often confusing, and disjointed thoughts into a more tangible, organized, and possibly reachable goal.

The vision board may also provide a space where a person can address their necessary life adjustments. As the board is created, their new role and its impact on their future may also be explored. Becoming future-focused facilitates meaning making: if a person can envision a future that they find exciting and hopeful, they may assign new meaning to the loss and how it could have created a positive change in their lives. In turn, it may further increase feelings of control, self-efficacy, and mastery.

GOAL

This process may address the 3rd and 4th Task of Mourning. Asking the client to explore their potential future after loss creates the potential for meaning making, instillation of hope, problem-solving, and creating goals to achieve future desires.

MATERIALS

Large paper (e.g., posterboard)

Markers/pens

Magazine/book clippings

Scissors

Glue

INSTRUCTION

Ask the client to consider their lives in the future (e.g., six months, one year, five years). What does this future look like? Where are they living? Working? What are they doing for fun? What would a fulfilling future mean to them? If they are feeling lost, you can start by asking them about the emotional aspects of their future first. How are you feeling in the future? This question can lead to what places, people, or activities have made them feel this way in the past. This exploration of the past can help give deeper insight and reflection into possible future goals. When they are ready, ask them to create a collage vision board that represents the future they would like to see themselves living.

POSSIBLE PROCESSING QUESTIONS AND PROMPTS

After your client completes their piece, ask them to reflect on what they created and consider the future life they have concretized in the visual form. The following questions may be used to further explore the process.

1. Can you tell me about your vision board and some of the elements you have included?

2. What are some things you would like to work toward that you have included?

3. What part of your vision board is most important to you? Why?

4. Which areas do you think will be the easiest to achieve? Most difficult? Most exciting? Most outside your comfort zone?

5. How did it feel to plan this new future?

6. How do you think considering your future in this way will change your actions and feelings now?

7. What steps do you think you can take to begin working toward this future? How does it feel to think about taking the steps you identified?

REFERENCES

American Psychiatric Association. (2022). *Diagnostic and Statistical Manual of Mental Disorders: DSM-5-TR*. American Psychiatric Association Publishing.

American Psychological Association. (2018). *Grief*. www.apa.org/topics/grief

American Psychological Association. (2023). *Trauma*. www.apa.org/topics/trauma

Bates-Maves, J. (2020). *Grief and Addiction*. Routledge. (See chapter 'Loss-Grief Addiction Model', pp.58–59.)

Beaumont, S. L. (2013). Art therapy for complicated grief: A focus on meaning-making approaches. *Canadian Art Therapy Association Journal, 26*(2), 1–7. https://doi.org/10.1080/08322473.2013.11415582

Beck, J., & Beck, A. (2011). *Cognitive Behavior Therapy: Basics and Beyond* (2nd edn). Guilford Press.

Bellini, S., Erbuto, D., Andriessen, K., Milelli, M., et al. (2018). Depression, hopelessness, and complicated grief in survivors of suicide. *Frontiers in Psychology, 9*. https://doi.org/10.3389/fpsyg.2018.00198

Blumer, H. (1969). *Symbolic Interactionism: Perspective and Method*. University of California Press.

Boelen, P. A., & Huntjens, R. J. (2008). Intrusive images in grief: An exploratory study. *Clinical Psychology & Psychotherapy, 15*(4), 217–226. https://doi.org/10.1002/cpp.568

Bolton, G. (2008). *Dying, Bereavement, and the Healing Arts*. Jessica Kingsley Publishers.

Bonanno, G. A. (2001). Grief and Emotion: A Social–Functional Perspective. In M. S. Stroebe, R. O. Hansson, W. Stroebe, & H. Schut (Eds.), *Handbook of Bereavement Research: Consequences, Coping, and Care* (pp.493–515). American Psychological Association. https://doi.org/10.1037/10436-021

Bowlby, J. (2008). *Attachment: Volume One of the Attachment and Loss Trilogy*. Vintage Digital.

Brier, N. (1999). Understanding and managing the emotional reactions to a miscarriage. *Obstetrics & Gynecology, 93*(1), 151–155. https://doi.org/10.1016/s0029-7844(98)00294-4

Burton, L., & Lent, J. (2016). The use of vision boards as a therapeutic intervention. *Journal of Creativity in Mental Health, 11*(1), 52–65. https://doi.org/10.1080/15401383.2015.1092901

Buzzell, L., & Chalquist, C. (2009). *Ecotherapy: Healing with Nature in Mind*. Sierra Club/Counterpoint.

Caruso-Teresi, M. (2017). The Women's Womb: Archetypal Imagery and Grieving Lost Self-Parts. In B. MacWilliam (Ed.), *Complicated Grief, Attachment, and Art*

Therapy: Theory, Treatment, and 14 Ready-to-Use Protocols (pp.293–305). Jessica Kingsley Publishers.

Charland, L. C. (2004). A madness for identity: Psychiatric labels, consumer autonomy, and the perils of the internet. *Philosophy, Psychiatry, & Psychology, 11*(4), 335–349. https://doi.org/10.1353/ppp.2005.0006

Chow, A. Y. (2009). Anticipatory anniversary effects and bereavement: Development of an integrated explanatory model. *Journal of Loss and Trauma, 15*(1), 54–68. https://doi.org/10.1080/15325020902925969

Conte, J. R. (2002). *Critical Issues in Child Sexual Abuse: Historical, Legal, and Psychological Perspectives*. Sage.

Cooper, R., Mishra, G., Hardy, R., & Kuh, D. (2009). Hysterectomy and subsequent psychological health: Findings from a British birth cohort study. *Journal of Affective Disorders, 115*(1–2), 122–130. https://doi.org/10.1016/j.jad.2008.08.017

Doka, K. J. (2002). *Disenfranchised Grief: New Directions, Challenges, and Strategies for Practice*. Research Press.

Doka, K. J. (2014). *Counseling Individuals with Life-Threatening Illness* (2nd ed.). Springer.

Farrington, D. P. (2014). *Labeling Theory: Empirical Tests*. Routledge.

Figley, C. R. (2013). *Traumatology of Grieving: Conceptual, Theoretical, and Treatment Foundations*. Taylor & Francis.

Figley, C. R., Bride, B. E., & Mazza, N. (1997). *Death and Trauma: The Traumatology of Grieving*. Routledge.

Freud, S. (2005). *On Murder, Mourning, and Melancholia*. Penguin Books.

Garti, D., & Bat Or, M. (2019). Subjective experience of art therapists in the treatment of bereaved clients. *Art Therapy, 36*(2), 68–76. https://doi.org/10.1080/0742165 6.2019.1609329

Gershfeld-Litvin, A. (2018). Women's experiences following mastectomy: Loss, grief, and meaning-reconstruction. *Illness, Crisis & Loss, 29*(3), 187–204. https://doi.org/10.1177/1054137318799046

Gesi, C., Carmassi, C., Cerveri, G., Carpita, B., Cremone, I. M., & Dell'Osso, L. (2020). Complicated grief: What to expect after the coronavirus pandemic. *Frontiers in Psychiatry, 11*. https://doi.org/10.3389/fpsyt.2020.00489

Gussak, D. (2019). *Art and Art Therapy with the Imprisoned: Re-creating Identity*. Routledge.

Gussak, D. E. (2015). *Art on Trial: Art Therapy in Capital Murder Cases*. Columbia University Press.

Harris, D. L. (2020). *Non-death Loss and Grief: Context and Clinical Implications*. Routledge.

Harris, N. (2002). Effective, short-term therapy: Utilizing finger labyrinths to promote brain synchrony. *Annals of the American Psychotherapy Association, 5*(5), 22–23.

Hinton, D. E., Peou, S., Joshi, S., Nickerson, A., & Simon, N. M. (2013). Normal grief and complicated bereavement among traumatized Cambodian refugees: Cultural context and the central role of dreams of the dead. *Culture, Medicine, and Psychiatry, 37*(3), 427–464. https://doi.org/10.1007/s11013-013-9324-0

Hinz, L. D. (2020). *Expressive Therapies Continuum: A Framework for Using Art in Therapy*. Routledge.

Hiyoshi, A., Berg, L., Saarela, J., Fall, K., et al. (2022). Substance use disorder and suicide-related behaviour around dates of parental death and its anniversaries:

A register-based cohort study. *The Lancet Public Health, 7*(8). https://doi.org/10.1016/s2468-2667(22)00158-x

Hunt, K. (2021). Bereavement behind bars: Prison and the grieving process. *Prison Service Journal,* 254, 17–23.

Jackson, L. L. (2020). *Signs: The Secret Language of the Universe.* Dial Press.

James, W. (1890/1918). *The Principles of Psychology. Vol.1 and Vol.2.* Henry Holt and Company.

Jones, S. J., & Beck, E. (2006). Disenfranchised grief and nonfinite loss as experienced by the families of death row inmates. *OMEGA – Journal of Death and Dying, 54*(4), 281–299. https://doi.org/10.2190/a327-66k6-p362-6988

Kaduson, H., Schaefer, C., & Aronson, J. (2001). *101 More Favorite Play Therapy Techniques, Volume 2.* Jason Aronson.

Kagin, S. L., & Lusebrink, V. B. (1978). The expressive therapies continuum. *Art Psychotherapy, 5*(4), 171–180. https://doi.org/10.1016/0090-9092(78)90031-5

Katon, J. G., Callegari, L. S., Bossick, A. S., Fortney, J., et al. (2020). Association of depression and post-traumatic stress disorder with receipt of minimally invasive hysterectomy for uterine fibroids: Findings from the U.S. Department of Veterans Affairs. *Women's Health Issues, 30*(5), 359–365. https://doi.org/10.1016/j.whi.2020.06.005

Kenney, J. S. (2002). Victims of crime and labeling theory: A parallel process? *Deviant Behavior, 23*(3), 235–265. https://doi.org/10.1080/01639620275561239

Kho, Y., Kane, R. T., Priddis, L., & Hudson, J. (2015). The nature of attachment relationships and grief responses in older adults: An attachment path model of grief. *PLOS ONE, 10*(10). https://doi.org/10.1371/journal.pone.0133703

Klass, D., Silverman, P. R., & Nickman, S. L. (1999). *Continuing Bonds: New Understandings of Grief.* Taylor & Francis.

Kokou-Kpolou, C. K., Fernández-Alcántara, M., & Cénat, J. M. (2020). Prolonged grief related to COVID-19 deaths: Do we have to fear a steep rise in traumatic and disenfranchised griefs? *Psychological Trauma: Theory, Research, Practice, and Policy, 12*(S1). https://doi.org/10.1037/tra0000798

Krakow, B., & Zadra, A. (2006). Clinical management of chronic nightmares: Imagery rehearsal therapy. *Behavioral Sleep Medicine, 4*(1), 45–70. https://doi.org/10.1207/s15402010bsm0401_4

Kübler-Ross. E. (1969). *On Death and Dying; Questions and Answers on Death and Dying; on Life After Death.* Quality Paperback Book Club.

Larson, L. (2017). The Memory Box. In B. MacWilliam (Ed.), *Complicated Grief, Attachment, and Art Therapy: Theory, Treatment, and 14 Ready-to-Use Protocols* (pp.188–203). Jessica Kingsley Publishers.

Latham, A. E., & Prigerson, H. G. (2004). Suicidality and bereavement: Complicated grief as psychiatric disorder presenting greatest risk for suicidality. *Suicide and Life-Threatening Behavior, 34*(4), 350–362. https://doi.org/10.1521/suli.34.4.350.53737

Leppert, P. C., Legro, R. S., & Kjerulff, K. H. (2007). Hysterectomy and loss of fertility: Implications for women's mental health. *Journal of Psychosomatic Research, 63*(3), 269–274. https://doi.org/10.1016/j.jpsychores.2007.03.018

Linehan, M. (2017). *DBT Skills Training Manual.* Guilford Press.

Lobb, E. A., Kristjanson, L. J., Aoun, S. M., Monterosso, L., Halkett, G. K., & Davies, A. (2010). Predictors of complicated grief: A systematic review of empirical studies. *Death Studies, 34*(8), 673–698. https://doi.org/10.1080/07481187.2010.496686

Loconto, D. G. (1998). Death and dreams: A sociological approach to grieving and identity. *OMEGA – Journal of Death and Dying, 37*(3), 171–185. https://doi.org/10.2190/gpy0-6vte-qv4m-tlnd

Lusebrink, V. B. (1987). Visual imagery: Its psychophysiological components and levels of information processing. *Imagination, Cognition and Personality, 6*(3), 205–218. https://doi.org/10.2190/q6jp-x6cw-mkah-faoh

Macdonald, A. J. (2011). *Solution-Focused Therapy: Theory, Research and Practice*. Sage.

MacWilliam, B. (Ed.). (2017). *Complicated Grief, Attachment, and Art Therapy: Theory, Treatment, and 14 Ready-to-Use Protocols*. Jessica Kingsley Publishers.

Marques, L., Bui, E., LeBlanc, N., Porter, E., et al. (2013). Complicated grief symptoms in anxiety disorders: Prevalence and associated impairment. *Depression and Anxiety, 30*(12), 1211–1216. https://doi.org/10.1002/da.22093

Martinez, N., Connelly, C. D., Perez, A., & Calero, P. (2021). Self-care: A concept analysis. *International Journal of Nursing Sciences*, 418–425. https://doi.org/10.1016/j.ijnss.2021.08.007

Mason, T. M., Tofthagen, C. S., & Buck, H. G. (2020). Complicated grief: Risk factors, protective factors, and interventions. *Journal of Social Work in End-of-Life & Palliative Care, 16*(2), 151–174. https://doi.org/10.1080/15524256.2020.1745726

Mead, G.H. (1964). On *Social Psychology*. University of Chicago Press.

Melhem, N. M., Day, N., Shear, M. K., Day, R., Reynolds, C. F., & Brent, D. (2004). Traumatic grief among adolescents exposed to a peer's suicide. *American Journal of Psychiatry, 161*(8), 1411–1416. https://doi.org/10.1176/appi.ajp.161.8.1411

Mittelman, M. S., Epstein, C., & Pierzchala, A. (2003). *Counseling the Alzheimer's Caregiver: A Resource for Health Care Professionals*. AMA Press.

Moore, R. L., & Havlick, M. J. (2001). *The Archetype of Initiation: Sacred Space, Ritual Process, and Personal Transformation: Lectures and Essays*. Xlibris Corp.

Morriss-Kay, G. M. (2010). The evolution of human artistic creativity. *Journal of Anatomy, 216*(2), 158–176. https://doi.org/10.1111/j.1469-7580.2009.01160.x

Moss, R. (2005). *The Dreamer's Book of the Dead: A Soul Traveler's Guide to Death, Dying, and the Other Side*. Destiny Books.

Neimeyer, R. A. (2001). *Meaning Reconstruction and the Experience of Loss*. American Psychological Association.

Neimeyer, R. A. (Ed.) (2012). *Techniques of Grief Therapy: Creative Practices for Counseling the Bereaved*. Routledge.

Neimeyer, R. A. (Ed.) (2016). *Techniques of Grief Therapy: Assessment and Intervention*. Routledge.

Nordell, J. (2021). *The End of Bias: A Beginning: The Science and Practice of Overcoming Unconscious Bias*. Metropolitan Books.

Novaco, R. W., & Chemtob, C. M. (1998). Anger and Trauma: Conceptualization, Assessment, and Treatment. In V. M. Follette, J. I. Ruzek, & F. R. Abueg (Eds.), *Cognitive-Behavioral Therapies for Trauma* (pp.162–190). Guilford Press.

Palgi, Y., Avidor, S., Shrira, A., Bodner, E., et al. (2018). Perception counts: The relationships of inner perceptions of trauma and PTSD symptoms across time. *Psychiatry, 81*(4), 361–375. https://doi.org/10.1080/00332747.2018.1485370

Peel, J. M. (2004). The labyrinth: An innovative therapeutic tool for problem solving or achieving mental focus. *The Family Journal, 12*(3), 287–291. https://doi.org/10.1177/1066480704264349

Pinto, P. R., McIntyre, T., Almeida, A., & Araújo-Soares, V. (2012). The mediating role of pain catastrophizing in the relationship between presurgical anxiety and acute postsurgical pain after hysterectomy. *Pain, 153*(1), 218–226. https://doi.org/10.1016/j.pain.2011.10.020

Plugg, C., & McCormick, D. (1997). *Walking a Path of Transformation: Using the Labyrinth as a Spiritual Tool.* https://eric.ed.gov/?id=ED414144

Potash, J. S., & Handel, S. (2012). Memory Boxes. In R. A. Neimeyer (Ed.), *Techniques of Grief Therapy: Creative Practices for Counseling the Bereaved* (pp.243–246). Routledge.

Rando, T. (1984). *Grief, Dying, and Death: Clinical Interventions for Caregivers.* Research Press.

Rando, T. (2000). *Clinical Dimensions of Anticipatory Mourning: Theory and Practice in Working with the Dying, their Loved Ones, and Their Caregivers.* Research Press.

Read, S. (2018). *Loss, Dying and Bereavement in the Criminal Justice System.* Routledge.

Rogers, J. E., & Feldman, J. (2007). Alternative Art Forms. In J. E. Rogers (Ed.), *The art of Grief: The Use of Expressive Arts in a Grief Support Group* (pp.239–257). Routledge.

Rosal, M. L. (2018). Cognitive-Behavioral Art Therapy. In J. A. Rubin (Ed.), *Approaches to Art Therapy: Theory and Technique* (pp.333–352). Routledge.

Russ, V., Stopa, L., Sivyer, K., Hazeldine, J., & Maguire, T. (2022). The relationship between adult attachment and complicated grief: A systematic review. *OMEGA – Journal of Death and DyingOmega (Westport)*, 003022282210831. https://doi.org/10.1177/00302228221083110

Russell, V. M., Baker, L. R., & McNulty, J. K. (2013). Attachment insecurity and infidelity in marriage: Do studies of dating relationships really inform us about marriage? *Journal of Family Psychology, 27*(2), 242–251. https://doi.org/10.1037/a0032118

Sagula, D., & Rice, K. G. (2004). The effectiveness of mindfulness training on the grieving process and emotional well-being of chronic pain patients. *Journal of Clinical Psychology in Medical Settings, 11*(4), 333–342. https://doi.org/10.1023/b:jocs.0000045353.78755.51

Scheinfeld, E., Gangi, K., Nelson, E. C., & Sinardi, C. C. (2021). Please scream inside your heart: Compounded loss and coping during the COVID-19 pandemic. *Health Communication, 37*(10), 1316–1328. https://doi.org/10.1080/10410236.2021.1886413

Schneider, K. J., Pierson, J. F., Bugental, J. F. T., & Aanstoos, C. M. (2015). *The Handbook of Humanistic Psychology: Leading Edges in Theory, Research, and Practice.* Sage.

Servaty-Seib, H. L., & Chapple, H. S. (2021). *Handbook of Thanatology: The Essential Body of Knowledge for the Study of Death, Dying, and Bereavement.* Routledge.

Seymour, A., & Treadon, C. (2022). Growing with Grief: An Art Therapy Curriculum to Prevent Complicated Bereavement. American Art Therapy Association. Minneapolis. https://at-institute.arttherapy.org/products/self-study-gm15-growing-with-grief-an-art-therapy-curriculum-to-prevent-complicated-bereavement

Shear, K., & Shair, H. (2005). Attachment, loss, and complicated grief. *Developmental Psychobiology, 47*(3), 253–267. https://doi.org/10.1002/dev.20091

Shear, M. K. (2012). Grief and mourning gone awry: Pathway and course of complicated grief. *Dialogues in Clinical Neuroscience, 14*(2). https://doi.org/10.31887/DCNS.2012.14.2/mshear

Shear, M. K. (2015). Complicated grief. *New England Journal of Medicine, 372*(2), 153–160. https://doi.org/10.1056/nejmcp1315618

Sieff, D. (2015). *Understanding and Healing Emotional Trauma.* Routledge.

Silove, D., Tay, A., Steel, Z., Tam, N., et al. (2017). Symptoms of post-traumatic stress disorder, severe psychological distress, explosive anger and grief amongst partners of survivors of high levels of trauma in post-conflict Timor-Leste. *Psychological Medicine, 47*(1), 149–159. https://doi.org/10.1017/S0033291716002233

Stroebe, M., & Schut, H. (1999). The dual process model of coping with bereavement: Rationale and description. *Death Studies, 23*(3), 197–224. https://doi.org/10.1080/074811899201046

Taylor, S. (2021). Transformation through loss and grief: A study of personal transformation following bereavement. *The Humanistic Psychologist, 49*(3), 381–399. https://doi.org/10.1037/hum0000172

Thompson, B. E., & Neimeyer, R. (2014). *Grief and the Expressive Arts: Practices for Creating Meaning.* Routledge.

Valle, M. F., Huebner, E. S., & Suldo, S. M. (2006). An analysis of hope as a psychological strength. *Journal of School Psychology, 44*(5), 393–406. https://doi.org/10.1016/j.jsp.2006.03.005

Van Gordon, W., Shonin, E., & Richardson, M. (2018). Mindfulness and nature. *Mindfulness, 9*(5), 1655–1658. https://doi.org/10.1007/s12671-018-0883-6

Van Lith, T. (2014). "Painting to find my spirit": Art making as the vehicle to find meaning and connection in the Mental Health Recovery Process. *Journal of Spirituality in Mental Health, 16*(1), 19–36. https://doi.org/10.1080/19349637.2013.864542

van Wielink, J., Wilhelm, L., & van Geelen-Merks, D. (2020). *Loss, Grief, and Attachment in Life Transitions: A Clinician's Guide to Secure Base Counseling.* Routledge.

Weiskittle, R., & Gramling, S. (2018). The therapeutic effectiveness of using visual art modalities with the bereaved: A systematic review. *Psychology Research and Behavior Management, 11*, 9–24. https://doi.org/10.2147/prbm.S131993

Worden, J. W. (2018). *Grief Counseling and Grief Therapy: A Handbook for the Mental Health Practitioner* (5th edn). Springer.

Wright, S. T., Kerr, C. W., Doroszczuk, N. M., Kuszczak, S. M., Hang, P. C., & Luczkiewicz, D. L. (2013). The impact of dreams of the deceased on bereavement. *American Journal of Hospice and Palliative Medicine, 31*(2), 132–138. https://doi.org/10.1177/1049909113479201

Yalom, I. D. (1980). *Existential Psychotherapy.* Basic Books.

Yalom, I. D. (2009). *Staring at the Sun: Overcoming the Terror of Death.* Jossey-Bass.

Yen, J.-Y., Chen, Y.-H., Long, C.-Y., Chang, Y., et al. (2008). Risk factors for major depressive disorder and the psychological impact of hysterectomy: A prospective investigation. *Psychosomatics, 49*(2), 137–142. https://doi.org/10.1176/appi.psy.49.2.137

Young, H., & Garrard, B. (2015). Bereavement and loss: Developing a memory box to support a young woman with profound learning disabilities. *British Journal of Learning Disabilities, 44*(1), 78–84. https://doi.org/10.1111/bld.12129

Yücel, D. E., van Emmerik, A. A. P., Souama, C., & Lancee, J. (2020). Comparative efficacy of imagery rehearsal therapy and prazosin in the treatment of trauma-related nightmares in adults: A meta-analysis of randomized controlled trials. *Sleep Medicine Reviews, 50*, 101248. https://doi.org/10.1016/j.smrv.2019.101248

Zisook, S., & Shear, K. (2009). Grief and bereavement: What psychiatrists need to know. *World Psychiatry, 8*(2), 67–74. https://doi.org/10.1002/j.2051-5545.2009.tb00217.x

SUBJECT INDEX

AUTHOR INDEX